Speak Gently: A Breast Cancer Journey

Speak Gently: A Breast Cancer Journey

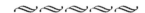

Diane Lanquetôt

Dalloway Press
ASHEVILLE, NC

Published by Dalloway Press, Asheville, NC

www.speakgently.com

Lanquetôt, Diane
Speak gently: a breast cancer journey/Diane Lanquetôt. — 1ˢᵗ ed.

p.   cm.

ISBN 978-0-692-54165-4

1. Memoirs and biographies. 2. Autobiography—Women authors.
3. Mothers and daughters. 4. Cancer & health. 5. Breast—Cancer—
Patients-—Family relationships. 6. Breast cancer patients' writings,
American. 7. Breast—Cancer—Poetry. 8. New England —Poetry.
 9. Rhode Island —Poetry. 10. Breast—Cancer—Treatment.
11. Chemotherapy. 12. Mastectomy—Autobiography. 13. Personal
narratives—American. 14. Grief and loss. 15. Gardening. I. Title.

for Mom

Merci

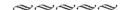

In 1959 my mother had a radical mastectomy at the age of 26. My sister Carol died of breast cancer on August 21, 2004. She was 45. My father died of lymphoma on October 29, 2009. He was 76.

After a layoff, I returned home to Rhode Island in 2011 to stay with my widowed mother for what was meant to be a temporary respite. On March 20, 2012, I was diagnosed with Stage II breast cancer at the age of 47. Twelve days later my mother was diagnosed with Stage III colon cancer.

We were treated at separate facilities, but shared this journey with the love and support of family and friends over the next ten months.

My mother died of breast cancer on February 8, 2013. She was 79.

MARCH

CAN'T SAY THAT I'M MOURNING MY BREASTS —

Maple bones rock —

Birdhouses swing —

— ONLY MY INTACT —

Wind, winds, enough to crack a —

Sun a bit higher, a bit stronger.

— MORE THAN MY BODY PARTS —

— *may* happen —

Maple bones quake —

Begin, begin (finish before you —

Today's mail, the heirloom seeds, experimental package from the Baker Creek catalog.

Sparrows sway, giddy carnival —

For the first time in my life I consider the sun's journey around the house (or house's journey around the sun) —

Cornucopia of pepper specks —

— dawn — day — dusk, window by window —

— tan slivers, shriveled paper dots —

" — *popular variety at the turn of the century* —

(enough to start a modest plantation —

— quake and resolve —

I line peat pots across the southern sills to maximize the weak winter sun.

— *may* happen —

I was so sorry to hear about your mother.

— *has* happened (finish before —

With deepest sympathy

germination = soil + water

In loving memory

+ sun + maniacal hovering

— glossy, colored pages, carrot crops dancing in my —

Baker Creek, Mansfield, Missouri (home of Laura Ingalls Wilder) —

Dwarf Siberian kale, 250 (!) seeds in the packet —

— cucumber groves —

Heirloom seeds blessed by Laura and Almanzo.

You can shed tears she is gone

Filtered water and seed starting mix; 'greenhouse' wrap across the tray on top of the warmish refrigerator.

Not seventy-two hours and twelve miracles in the night, stalks tipped with four oval leaves.

You can shed tears —

I fawn and stare, anxious —

Never assume the person <u>cannot hear</u>; hearing is the last of the senses to be —

Begin, begin (finish before —

smile because she has

I sat bedside, holding her hand, chest rising and falling—

— knick-knacks, sunny sills stripped of miniature Elizabethan houses; lamp-posts; Victorians; cottages by-the-sea; pewter pitcher and salt shaker ...

— agape; oxygen machine grumbling on the floor against the —

... small colored bottles (blue in the side room, reds and golds in the den) that match the wallpapers —

> "— *Russian variety produces leaves that are only slightly frilled* —"

At the base of some of the bottles are dead flies.

Pink Cup, Blue Cup —

Southern sills for maximum —

I rinse them with water to flush out the bodies.

— ceramic dishes she collected over —

We were made to choke down sewer water, sadistic quantities for reasons neither of us quite fathomed at the onset.

*"Direct-seeded or started and transplanted
before the last frost."*

I thought to flush our systems, our kidneys —

Dwee-buh-dee —

These *Boston Pickling* cucumbers date back to 1880.

Dwee-buh-dee —

Slim green petals open-mouthed —

— insult of filthy, month-old snow through the window.

Wrens? Robins?

Dwee-buh-dee — dwee-buh-dee —

Sparrows?

What sayest thou, mon ami?

How do you like the new house, the snazzy gold condo
beside your homely wooden —

Dwee-buh-dee — dwee-buh-dee (dissecting this affront —
'gentrification' —

I soon apprehended that the Waking Hour sip-pee, sip-
pee, sip-pee, Nocturnal pee-pee-pee sewer water regimen

was to mitigate the as never before experienced, and
hope never to again —

Dinnertime, pecking the hard brown ground for buried—

sorrow at this sad

Solitary someone high in the —

Rip Van Woodchucks plot garden raids, biding the
calendar, yet I persist, juggling tippy peat pots on sills
and cookie sheets —

— *"last frost date"*?

Flat of Italy onions push up tiny grasses.

I press aluminum foil onto the trays to concentrate the
weak window light.

Consult *Farmers Almanac*?

Dwee-dwee-dwee —

— from every source: number of days, hours, minutes to
germinate, cultivate, water, fertilize, mulch, 'harden',
space, transplant, weed (how anything has ever
managed, since the beginnings of —

'Red-breasted Nuthatch'? *'Northern Mockingbird'*? (battered
bird guide from the sunporch rack —

Dwee-buh-dee —

Bugs writhe beneath panes and knock at screens —

a bright soul

Fat fur slithers through the yard on a clover mission,
munching, then gorging on the wide open —

Birds <u>do</u> pollinate — seeds straight through their —

Why me.

Puppet or Muppet on the wall grazing chive tips —

Why not me (not forty-eight hours —

On the loss of your Mother

Tipping shower: (1) wads choking the drain (2) tangled,
unrinsable strands pasted on my chest, scars, arms and
neck.

With the orange paper scissors I clipped as close to my
head as I could, filling the sink with brown waves.

I found her electric razor under the sink and buzzed up
and down, over the ears and behind, using the double
mirror to refine my stubble scalp.

You have a nice head.

We did, in fact, smile.

More satisfying than television.

I stroked my stubble, fingered my *furred fontanel* like a cat for the next six months.

Can I catch them growing if I stare hard enough?

NB: whirring scalp, dull 'cap' sensation(?)

— intermittent —

A thousand times a day to the pots on their trays, on the sills, lifting, rearranging, moving one a millimeter closer to the sun as shade encroaches.

comfort in special memories

Tippy peat pots on kitchen, living room, sunporch, bedroom, computer room sills: *Genovese* basil; *Santa Fe Grande* pepper; *Giant of Italy* parsley; *Boston Pickling* cucumber ...

soothing to your soul

... *Slo-Bolt* cilantro; *Serrano Tampiqueno*; *Gotte Jaune d'Or* lettuce; *Black Beauty* zucchini —

Cukes salute their One Week Birthday — nearly two inches tall!

memories and all she

Vivid leaves I must stop myself from —

in my prayers

— neither colored nor cut for many months) with enough strands remaining. I trimmed the white hair with the same chunky orange paper scissors, blunt around the ears and across her neck, coaxing a style.

Why not —

She seemed pleased.

Why the hot peppers are so sluggish to sprout — *Serrano Tampiqueno* in New England spring, wind chills well below —

the one who loved you from the beginning

Clear calm sky and a walk — my walk — briskly, near normally, incapable six months ago without palpitations and fear of heart attack; dragging of feet underwater; avoidance of all but the most baby inclinations.

wishing you

Peat pots — pleasant woody or woodsy drafts of —

One Mass Daily in Perpetuity

Why not (not forty-eight hours —

For the first time in months, decent sun returns and warms the pots.

Boston Picklings stand tall, wings to the pane.

Genovese basil sets cloverish shoots.

> *"I HAVE BEEN SAVING THIS CARD FOR <u>YEARS</u>, WAITING FOR THE OCCASION SIGNIFICANT ENOUGH TO PART WITH IT."*

Flat of Italy onion filaments, looped closed, snap free and stand solo, taller than imagined, in somewhat shock.

> *"SO THE BLUE POODLE COMES TO YOU IN THIS SURREAL MOMENT - WHATEVER COMFORT AND ENCOURAGEMENT CAN BE BORNE ACROSS MILES AND YEARS FOR THE HONORING OF YOUR BREASTS AND THEIR DEPARTURE."*

Hours screen-benumbed, trying to glean some of the tricks of this method called 'lasagna', which might have been designed for seniors, or those with diminishing capacities to bend, kneel, stoop, lift, or wield a heavy shovel.

Recognizing Signs & Symptoms of End of Life

One makes a 'lasagna' of carbon-rich layers and nitrogen-rich layers on top of even the crummiest, weediest, mossiest, godforsaken patch of undeveloped yard and — POOF—

PHYSICAL SIGNS

(Would anyone but a crazy person hand-water forty peat pots with a toy-like mister of filtered, room temperature tap water to the point of arthritic sensations in both —

smile and kindness

... layers of soaked newspapers; layers of 'green' (grass clippings, spent plants, fruit and vegetable scraps, coffee grounds, tea bags, seaweed); layers of 'brown' (shredded leaves, twigs, pine needles, straw, newspaper) until the spongy mess breaks down over time into 'black gold'...

Hurrah — *Santa Fe* peppers have popped at last with the help of a heating pad, teeny —

> *"A CHANGE OF SCENE MIGHT BE A NICE BREAK - IT'S STILL COLD (FOR HERE) BUT CLEAR AND SUNNY."*

Scavenger hunt for the 'brown': garbage bag of crisp wintered leaves from woods at the top of the hill, convenient wind-blown mounds (but for beer bottle shards) against the low stone wall.

> *"YOU AND YOUR FAMILY HAVE BEEN THROUGH SUCH —"*

— glass chunks with gloved fingers (am I an idiot?)

> *"I'M SURE YOU LIKED THEM."*

21

I secure the crackling 'lasagna' fodder in the trunk, then hang the bag on a peg in the shed to await further rumination —

How this can be —

— cogitation —

At Resurrection, unable to complete my six laps (not for a year now), fatigue approaching lap number —

> *"I'M SURE IT WILL BE VERY STRANGE AND SAD NOT TO—"*

— post-surgical protrusions or 'dog ears' in the center of my chest without clear explanation from anyone as to —

— saliva — lashes — pubes —

> *"I HOPE YOU HEAL QUICKLY."*

To do: call Caron and order year for the stone: 2-0-1-3

— nose hair —

Lap number —

BODY TEMPERATURE (increasingly cool to the —

— insurance; bank; pension; Medicare; medical bills (hundreds of disconnected companies presenting charges under the most —

" — water with care so as not to soak roots, risk rot —"

— pamphlets; papers; brochures; carbon copies; nurses' notes; summaries; equipment invoices in a box top on the massive desk —

Lap number —

"Avoid the leaves."

 The loam has contracted several inches since the rain, producing a caved-in appearance as though she literally had <u>rolled over</u> —

— lashes — brows —

> THANKS FOR THE BEAUTIFUL ZEN CARD AND
> ESPECIALLY THE BRONTË ARTICLE. IT'S A VERY
> MAGICAL PLACE. I'VE BEEN TO HAWORTH TWICE
> AND WOULD LOVE TO GO AGAIN IN THIS
> LIFETIME.

Squirming, trying to settle in my lap, her toddler head smashed my scar and gave me an electric shock.

> OUT OF THE HOSPITAL MONDAY AND
> PROGRESSING WELL, MEETING WITH <u>HER</u>
> ONCOLOGIST ON TUESDAY.

(I made a mental note to pull out the cheap spongy prosthetic next visit.)

— approaching lap number —

— 'center of balance' right away, slow revolution down
the hospital corridor (six pounds in three hours?)

— FOR THE CHEER AND THE HUMBLE —

Quite the dive!

HOME ANY MINUTE AFTER HER 10-DAY
HOSPITAL VENTURE DOWN THE RABBIT —

"Big Clock, Lil' Clock", she clapped and called them.

Black Beauty zuke off the upper sill. I sweep the soil into
my palm, direct it back in the peat pot, and rearrange the
seedling.

Filtered sun, through screen and window —

The green shoot still wears its husk like a little hat.

— widest section of the circle — lap number —

— *will be fine* — sip of water from my own glass —

Two-week *Boston Pickling* birthday; first fuzzy, notched
'true' leaves emerge after the embryonic *cotyledons*.

— *all is well* —

Giant of Italy parsley spills over her peat box in jailbreak.

24

Basil waits on heat, ogling the window box spring mix, indistinguishable profusion of *Monstrueux de Viroflay* spinach, *Dwarf Siberian* kale, *Gotte Jaune d'Or* lettuce —

Growth — daily —

— that human hair is 'good for gardens' and can be composted or strewn 'around borders' to deter critters, so I put the clippings from the most recent trim of my permy chemo curls (a brown fluff ball that looks suspiciously alive) into a plastic bag and leave it on the back of the toilet for the time —

Dwarf Siberian kale 'true' leaves, jagged borders with neat networks of veins —

Not long — three weeks after the first infusion?

— *a nice shaped head,* she said.

— as inevitable, we thumbed through both print and electronic versions of the American Cancer Society TLC (Tender Loving Care) catalog and ordered advance terrycloth turbans — a bright red and a dark blue for me, a baby blue and a pink for her —

— *furred fontanel* —

I would wear these snug turbans for the next six months in alternation, removing them only to shower or sleep.

My mother, who retained most of her naturally sparse hair throughout treatment, wore neither, preferring her favorite pink Red Sox cap.

We also bought cheap wigs from the same catalog — mine an ash pixie, hers a snappy —

warm and intelligent

I wore the wig to two or three infusions before folding it back in the plastic and stuffing it in the closet.

The peat pots are beginning to crumble.

She wore hers on the one occasion, Thanksgiving at my aunt's, beside whom she posed, smiling, on a couch, the last picture she would ever —

RESTLESSNESS (repetitive motions —

 — though I did creep there often, to my specific subheadings, to find out if any 'sisterfriends' around the country, around the world ever had — or —

> WHATEVER IT IS, I HOPE EVERYONE CAN HAVE THE SAME SPIRIT AND NOT LET THIS POISON THEIR LIVES TOO MUCH.

 — and what — would very likely —

 — nowhere near warm enough to put them in the ground.

helps and heals

Daffodils — suddenly — against the wall (and she, not here —

APRIL

*"We are sparks, we are shadows, we are pollen,
which the next wind will carry away."*

OLIVE SCHREINER, STORY OF AN AFRICAN FARM

— room to room, drawer to drawer, shelf to shelf —

— HER SAD SHOCKED FACE ALL DAY —

— her affinity for horizontal stripes —

— *furred* —

I discover this bit of trivia sorting through piles of polos,
knits, sweaters —

— saliva and no ability to produce saliva day after day,
week after week.

Wonder of perennials — better than any —

When I woke in the mornings, deliberate Tin Man efforts
to lubricate my rusted mouth, tongue scraping teeth,
moving my jaw in and out in pumplike —

— field glasses through the window —

— bloody clots wrapped around black spikes of nose hair—

My nose ran on and —

— clots and spikes — clots and —

— blood and clots on tissues for what seemed like —

I pull a soft blue sweater ringed with red and yellow stripes over my head.

The fourth *Black Beauty* zuke seed has erupted at last in her pot, heaving soil on either side, tricked via heating pad into thinking she's moved to Florida.

— clots and spikes until the nose was fully deforested.

This, too, exacerbated Parch Mouth —

— coats in the closet, Crayola box of jackets for every season — green, blue, black, red, yellow —

Into the collapsed garbage bag: underwear; bras; yellowed, ancient prosthesis; unworn wig; toothbrush —

Blue theme — her blue eyes —

I help the *Black Beauty* zukes shed their sticky husks by picking them off with my fingernail.

A riot of coats? A murder of coats?

White residue — mildew(?) — on some leaves.

SUBJECT: HIGHLY UNPLEASANT NEWS

Flock? Bevy? Covey?

Sixteen *Boston Pickling* seedlings, 100% germination, in eight pots across the sunny sills — my unintentional Cucumber Farm.

No. One for the bugs; one for the squirrels; disease; woodchucks —

Or as *Pa* was wont to sing each spring:

> *One for the gopher*
>
> *Two for the gopher*
>
> *Three for the gopher*
>
> *Four don't go fur.*

Called Caron, ordered the 2-0-1-3 for the —

Touched that she mailed me packets of wildflower seeds,
but how to squeeze flowers beside edibles in the limited
real estate of the back yard.

— has returned in the usual places, though the hair on
my head is not my hair but a crop of imposter permy
curls which is, as I've read, not at all —

— GENETIC TESTS — BACK NEXT —

Three weeks prior, another train whistle (premonition?)
blast in the middle of the night, though she'd insisted she
couldn't remember —

THANKS AGAIN FOR YOUR THOUGHTS AND
GOOD —

Pristine, serene Resurrection as personal walking track,
wide circular laps around Mémère, Pépère, Dad, and now
Mom in their plot by the chapel.

The air, too, is breezier, fresher than anywhere in the —

— PEACE WITH THIS IF IT IS MY —

DISORIENTATION (time, place identity)

— mourners at two or three any time of day. Widows
and widowers disembark from sedate, polished vehicles
and pick their way through the turf, between the stones,
to their future graves.

Daughters. Sons. Couples.

They may leave a bouquet, but mostly they stand and stare.

I pass and watch them watching the grave.

OF COURSE I DON'T MIND YOUR PRAYERS.

Dwee-buh-dee quank-quank in the bare branches —

Stare in disbelief.

Lilacs in the upper yard begin —

CONGESTION (gurgling sounds)

— *quank-quank*—

The gravediggers open plots with a small backhoe or 'Caterpillar'(?). They roll back the sod and scoop a great mound of fill into the back of the truck until it can be returned to the hole.

Was it suicide — *Black Beauty's* flight from the sill, unwilling to face the sun and put down roots —

The heavy truck drives over wooden boards placed end to end and tamped into place, a path from 'road' to grave to preserve the golfish grass.

Did he resent my packing the soil again and dousing on water, letting in light —

Too, too perfect green —

Check plot — see if grass has started to —

INCONTINENCE (loss of bladder and/or bowel control)

Why not natural decomposition, a là linen-shroud Jesus,
as opposed to sealed steel —

Forsythia begins to brilliant along the driveway.

— stacked on the hutch because I don't know what to —

— *may* happen —

I pass the seventeen-year-old's grave at the far end, his
framed portrait against the stone.

— *has* happened —

Mother? – sister? – aunts? – grandmother? – girlfriend?
visit often, in different combinations.

In decent weather they spread a blanket on the ground.

**Sleeping more frequently will occur with or without
medication.**

Quank-quank —

— from my experimental garden are most vulnerable:
swirl of blue jays; blur of squirrels along the chain link
fences; twitchy Tan Bunny in the lilac; marauder-in-chief,
Mr. Woodchuck 'en famille' —

— *will* happen —

Twelve feet outside the bathroom window in the small, abandoned, dilapidated 19th century cemetery is the main 'chuck burrow entrance, a large hole beside a much larger hill of pale dug dirt, rocks, broken twigs and dried leaves.

"... garden hose to tossing in laxatives, has been tried at one time or another to rid these — "

Mr. W hesitates behind the shower curtain, then slithers off the wall in search of something edible on the dried brown lawn of scrubby weeds and moss islands; hopeful spikes of green.

Must I be quite so ruthless?

SIGNS & SYMPTOMS: Recognizing Signs & Symptoms of —

Instructed to snip one of the seedlings from each peat pot, the 'weaker' of the pair, though both appear equally healthy (roots 'entwine', 'robbing nutrients', 'six inches apart minimum' —

Clouds and cools, spring and unspringlike —

Whither, whither doth this subterranean burrow wind?

Dipping and curving through skulls and bones that rode horses and buggies; swung lanterns; churned butter; read and wrote by candlelight —

Mission: **With compassion and skill we care for people living with serious illness —**

Rains and winds, droughts and heat waves, hurricanes and blizzards, until one by one the few dozen stones toppled and cracked, crumbled on the root-strewn ground and no one came to right them.

— green and blue long-sleeved striped shirt (over her head, bandaged lesion on her back, arms through the holes —

Come summertime, weeds and brush and poison ivy will choke off all views to the interior.

— *you don't need a bra, leave it off* — though unthinkable (prosthesis tucked away —

Last. The last shirt she —

Long ago we read the old timey inscriptions.

— those who are dying, and all who are —

Our rubber-coated homeruns bounced into the brush from the other side of Bartlett Street.

"... dismantle the garden bite by frustrating — "

Neighbors hurled dog poo into the big green jungle with
abandon.

Lopsided; unbalanced; one sagging breast, one flat scar;
first time I ever saw —

The hearse glided through the traffic light.

I laid my head down —

Maybe —

I clip the stems at soil level with the kitchen shears.

— sensation suspect, as the beginnings of —

I drop the four snipped seedlings in a Mason jar of water
to see if they might revivify, sprout roots or tendrils
through the clear glass.

Waiting on the true —

— not terrible, to be sure, though the stubble came to
grate a bit against pillows.

— evening watching tennis — many, many hours of —

Four laps would be an accomplishment as stamina
continues to —

Tennis (vicarious speed, zest, zip) trance —

One year ago today my breasts, one ill and one well —

— vaginal ache —

— armpit tugs —

— blotch of never seen rash directly below my —

Back and forth across the net —

"Big Clock, Lil' Clock" —

— of the long-range plan, a project to be completed in
three years, I cannot wrap my head around —

Emboldened, I plot a follow-up assassination, the runt of
her three Christmas cacti in the sunporch, coveting
planter and stand for herbs or greens.

— thrumming skull —

Bolts of Christmas red — thirty, forty blooms out of
season —

How this can be —

— many, many sets of pajamas. My aunt requests a pair.

After my sister's death we gathered in her bedroom and
distributed her discriminating boots, coats, tops, gloves.

How —

For years I wore her Eskimo-warm fuchsia parka, though with our height difference the sleeves were comically long.

Shock of butter-yellow forsythia along the driveway —

Her delicious purple dress shirt never failed to receive compliments. I took a leather coat, too, and eight years later returned it, unworn, to my niece on her 18th birthday.

Robins rage against the feeble, anemic lawn.

A sister-in-law shared her shoe size and took several pairs.

Even my mother took some blazers and a few —

How, then, to carry out —

— her spindly old basil in the plastic pot: (1) dash to the cemetery (2) dump contents down the burrow —

Did he not, too — Henry David — vow to catch and "eat one raw" —

Severing at the surface seems more humane than overturning the whole still breathing, pot-shaped, roots-exposed carcass.

I wear gloves for the poison ivy (and possible sumac) along the edges of the cemetery wall.

A year ago *this* —

— distinct sharp burning in the left forearm, of which I tried to alert the nurses (they even lifted my mask so I could speak) — recovery cubicle.

Two seconds. Not like sleeping or dreaming.

Daffodils, suddenly, against the —

No sensation of time having passed or having been in any way a participant.

Mr. W in the neighbor's yard this morning, trawling for dewy clover.

Single stems *do* thrive in peat pots, no longer competing—

No pain.

Wind *does* whistle though cliché. Maybe nor'easter, were there precipitation and temperatures forty degrees cooler.

Maybe some fallen limb, nature's blow to the back of Mr. W's little skull (poked out of the burrow, nosy —

> "... I caught a glimpse of a woodchuck stealing
> across my path, and felt a strange thrill of
> savage delight, and was strongly tempted to
> seize and devour him raw ..."

Dr. D— held my hands and rubbed them while his colleague rocked me forward to inject an additional potion into my spine.

Maybe —

Patches of whitish, mold-like fuzz have appeared on the sides of the dampened pots; seedlings indifferent.

Clandestine cactile decapitation —

The whitish fuzz seems to disappear as the pots dry.

Dr. D— tried to dissuade me —

Disposable gloves to perform —

Not half an hour before the procedure, in the pre-op cubicle, Dr. D— professed ignorance of the plan to remove *both* breasts.

He tried to dissuade me (another surgery? important meeting?), though we'd discussed this option at our consult, weeks prior, to which he'd agreed was entirely—

<u>BILATERAL MASTECTOMY</u>

— and his office had forwarded all the necessary —

... blah blah...

He said I'd experience not just <u>this</u> but <u>that</u> ... and much more than twice the —

... blah blah blah ...

BILATERAL MASTECTOMY

— many removed in his long career, enough to build a small mountain —

... blah blah ... "highly curable" ... blah blah ... blah blah ... blah ... "these days" ... blah blah ...

BILATERAL MASTECTOMY WITH RIGHT AXIAL NODE DISSECTION, April 18th, 2012, at —

Later, when the steri-strips that hadn't fallen off were taken off by a nurse, the right scar appeared markedly neater.

... blah ...

The left — healthy side — flared wide out to the corner of the armpit, with a puffier 'dog ear' flap left behind in the middle of my chest.

... blah ... blah blah ...

(Rush job? Resident?)

— asymmetrical, and right far neater than left.

(Chemo-noia?)

One week to May and still wearing her (perfectly functional) black winter coat to walk Resurrection.

"... not that I was hungry then, except for that wildness which he represented."

They will send someone out to ensure the font is matched with the extant etching, then contact me when the job is completed.

Raised, red, dime-sized growth along the left shoulder blade —

— this on my stomach above the belly button.

Beginnings of —

Adenocarcinoma that signaled the beginning of —

We took the most expedient dermatologist referral (a visiting nurse happened to peek down her shirt and made an appointment on the spot), a ratty-looking office across from the mall. She maneuvered very well on the icy driveway with the walker, a rare foray since the broken hip.

NONE OF THIS IS FUN. MOSTLY IT'S DISGUSTING.

I helped her remove her coat and lean her cane against the chair in the waiting room.

— faded, slightly scaly, patch of —

She sliced it off and put it in a dish extended by her assistant, *no, not related to* —

I stare at the pots on the sills, as if I could catch them —

— *no, not related* —

Two rows of wide wooden planks, like playing cards, overlapping, from grave to road.

— eczema? —

> — NOW CARING FOR HER <u>THIRD</u> IMMEDIATE FAMILY MEMBER (AND SHE MORE FUNCTIONAL THAN I) AS WE RACE (OR WALK SLOWLY) EACH OTHER TO THE —

Zuke pots crumble, though frost danger —

— fuzzy mold-growth from the sides of the pots with a tissue —

Daffodils, resolute, along the back wall —

> OPERATED ON AS I WRITE TO HAVE A LEFT HIP REPLACEMENT. CRASHED TO THE KITCHEN FLOOR.

6:32 AM. I thread my way through the basement to the driveway for the newspaper, past my parents' assistive devices, stacked and leaned among boxes, tools, and snow shovels: the white plastic shower bench; three folded walkers; two gray canes ...

43

MERRY CHRISTMAS TO US ALL.

... and a whi-i-i-te plastic raised toilet seat —

— 'nest' in her azaleas, she says, three hundred miles
south, where the cardinals camouflage.

**The most appropriate interventions at this stage are comfort-
enhancing measures.**

MAY

*"At present nothing is possible except
to extend the area of sanity little by little."*

GEORGE ORWELL, <u>1984</u>

Miracle sun —

Maple buds — lilacs —

    — INSTANT MENOPAUSE FOR A FUN-FILLED
    BONUS —

Brown scarred yard —

— playing card boards, end to end, to preserve the
pristine —

Flowers on graves; flags on veterans' for Memorial Day
— my father's (plucked up and planted down every
other—

— to simply —

The scar cream was called 'My Girls'.

— disappear —

I baked an appleberry pie while we waited and set it on a rack on the kitchen table. Med techs carried her though the front door on a stretcher, blue winter coat draped across her chest beneath the safety straps.

Growth — daily — visual inspection —

Wheels clanked and scraped the linoleum.

SLEEPING (increasing amount of time sleeping, appear to be uncommunicative or unresponsive —

Difficult to distinguish the jumble of salad sprouts in the indoor window box but arugula may be the grassier spears, not the shorter, more cloverish —

— penultimate full (could we have — could we —

They positioned her gently in her favorite chair in the sunporch.

Boo-wee — boo-wee —

One of the med-techs jammed a winter boot from the boot tray beneath each leg to prevent the chair from rocking or pitching forward.

— from the highest — *boo-wee* —

Splash of yellow against the wall. Glow of bright —

Growth — daily —

Quank—quank —

Blooms do "toss their heads in sprightly dance" —

The hospice nurse assured it was *okay to doze* and she
nodded off, chin upon green striped polo —

> — *gazed — and gazed — but little thought —*

— morphine and eye drops (not for eyes, we discovered),
among other medical —

— first pair of 'true' leaves after the *cotyledons* —

**USE 4 DROPS SUBLINGUALLY EVERY 4
HOURS AS NEEDED**

Armada? Sixty years of coats on hangers in the hall.

... *metronidazole* (Flagyl); *amlodipine* (Norvasc); *nebivolol*
(Bystolic); *rivaroxaban* (Xarelto); *sacchararomyces boulardii*
(Florastor); *atorvastatin* (Lipitor); *acetaminophen* ...

Black blazer she took from my sister's closet before the
funeral —

We put morsels of someone's leftover chicken in a tiny
Pyrex dish, fit for a baby. She wrapped her swollen
fingers around the adaptive fork and insisted she could—

... *ondansetron* HCl (Zofran) ; *morphine sulfate; lorazepam* (Ativan); *atropine sulfate ophthalmic solution* ...

In the brief window of appetite post-chemo, appleberry pie, made with apples, blueberries and raspberries, had become our new favorite.

Quank-quank —

<u>EVERY 4 HOURS</u>

— even smaller Pyrex cup with two bites of appleberry pie. *Yum*, she said, then put the fork on the tray, exhausted, her very last —

"What look like two leaves will appear."

— our accumulated mini-pharmacy, with some anti-nausea (*ondansetron*) and sedative (*lorazepam*) overlap, plastic bags of orange plastic bottles, opaque white bottles, boxes of tablets, in the top middle drawer of the hutch for 'responsible' (police department?) disposal at some future future.

ENCOURAGED TO SEE HAIR IN PLACES I'VE NOT SEEN —

Some of the bulkier ones (*Florastor* and the foul, PTSD *nystatin* mouthwash) I wedge in the side panel beside candles, ribbons, and bits of wrapping paper, and slam the door quickly like a stewardess.

Boo-wee — boo-wee —

At the highly ranked hospital where I'd been transferred and awaited a second port surgery (the first resulted in a partially collapsed lung), two women hovered by my bed. One stabbed me — tail on donkey — in the gross vicinity of what may or may not have been a vein (artery?) in my left forearm.

Boo-wee — boo-wee —

A geyser of red splashed the bedsheet.

Boo-wee — boo-wee —

The procedure was deemed a 'success' and the area hastily bandaged, taped and connected to a line.

The bloodied sheet was folded over on itself and tucked under the rail.

Biddle-biddle —

I showed the deep and hugebruised tenderness to one of the nurses — *it'll heal —*

Quank—quank —

— sore, sore for some weeks afterward — more than any other invasive (her veins, too, purple, rippled welts after every —

They gotcha good, said my phlebotomist at the clinic.

Vial after vial — enough to fill a water pitcher by summer's end.

They were able to ferret out the tiniest, well-pricked veins in the crook of my left arm with minimal — *small pinch* — discomfort, calmly and cheerfully.

— *sera* — *sera* —

I could see them following, silently acknowledging, my bi-weekly progress (regress): lush brunette to bald red turban; contacts to glasses; robust form to slow-motion weakling —

— *not an invalid* (adaptive rubber fork grip, appleberry bites —

'Dueling' clinics, mine with the (arguably) more —

Over time I preferred the blue terrycloth turban as less conspicuous than the red.

I did walk on the sidewalk, but so slowly that anyone accompanying me sailed ahead without much —

INTO THE QUE SERA, SERA MODE.

She wore her pink Red Sox cap and nothing —

— imagine befriending in another lifetime, my oncology nurse, C—

They were all good sports to match my plodding gait.

Over four months of infusions we chatted easily, about
her trip to Morocco, buying bags of saffron at the spice
bazaar, and how the airlines lost —

— burning, stinging in the armpit where old scar meets
new scar at a 45 degree angle —

I clip my Jerry-curl afro-mullet as it sprouts, and put the
rodent-like clippings in a Ziploc bag on the back of the
toilet.

'Coyote urine capsules' will repel any bothersome —

I laid my head on her chest —

I'm right behind you —

— ammonia (or urine) soaked rag stuffed in the burrow
hole —

Maybe it won't happen to you.

TURNED THE CORNER ON #10 THIS WEEK.

I laid my head on —

JUST TWO MORE FOR HER.

Haphazard spring sun through the closed —

Maybe it won't —

Black Beauty zukes sprawl, eager —

Must harden the babes soon, wean them off filtered water; perfect calm; rotated light sources; lovingly misted foliage —

Maybe, maybe —

Ammonia or <u>urine</u> down the hole!?

SHE ENJOYED HER BIRTHDAY AND ALL THE CALLS FROM EVERYONE.

— sprayed against my thigh six, seven, eight, nine times a—

Maybe —

(pubeless thoroughfare—

— against my thigh, sprayed down my —

— ten, eleven, twelve times a —

— **cool, moist washcloth on the forehead may increase physical** —

— *sera — sera —*

<u>USE 4 DROPS</u> —

— right behind you —

Monet golds, greens, yellows on the very tips —

— pubic tenderness —

Quank-quank —

No matter how I contorted, contorted and tried to
redirect the stream —

Bumblebee knock-knocks against the pane —

— twelve, thirteen times a —

— thigh, sprayed down my —

Also, the full body 'facial', the sloughing off. Even the
stubborn, impossible callus on the bottom of my foot
disappeared.

— again take for granted a not-so-simple —

White horizontal stripes bisected my fingernails in clear
demarcation; I did not lose any.

— golds, greens —

— cuts and infections with my nonexistent white —

Pale white tongue equaled plummeting danger zone.

Waiting, waiting on numbers —

Her lesion continued to ooze blood post-biopsy and did not seem to heal. We called the dermatologist — *this is normal.*

— yellows —

I gave myself a ferocious bloody paper cut ripping the plastic off her *Martha Stewart Living* —

> "... infections are a major cause of morbidity and mortality in patients who are *neutropenic* —"

— *normal* —

— thick, desperate layers of the same Neosporin© I applied daily to the dime-sized lesion on her —

Bills; junk; subscriptions; bills; bills; bills; confounding, multi-paged Medicare statements ...

Mr. W suns himself like a movie star on the cemetery wall.

— muscle weakness such that I had to raise and lower myself to and from the toilet using the vanity for leverage—

— *this is normal* —

The clipped *Boston Pickling* seedlings, started in the Mason jar, have proven to be an interesting hydroponic experiment, root hairs dangling, submerged, from each of the four stems.

What he does all day, guarding his entrance —

BEST STRATEGY IS NOT TO LOOK IN THE
MIRROR.

— as expected, though we could both eat white pasta with tomato sauce, the acidic tomatoes. Salad dressing also cut through.

What you do all day, passing mirrors —

Chronic bad taste in the mouth.

Train-track stitches, lines of looped, black thread-gut held my —

Even water tasted like sewage.

FAINTING EPISODE WAS A —

Coffee became repulsive, causing real panic, though she was able to drink her morning cup if decaffeinated.

FAINTING EPISODE WAS A COMBINATION OF
SLEEP DEPRIVATION, EXTREME EXHAUSTION
AFTER TRYING TO STAND AND SHOWER —

Chocolate repulsive.

— PTSD FROM LOOKING AT THE GRUESOME
INCISIONS AND FLAT, WEIRD, CONCAVE CHEST

IN THE MIRROR FOR THE FIRST TIME AFTER
TAKING OFF THE DRESSINGS —

I tried switching to tea but couldn't choke hot caffeinated tea in the morning.

— NOT EATING, TAKING WEIRD MEDS, MAKING
BAD DECISIONS BECAUSE I WAS SEMI-
DELIRIOUS.

Herbal was out. Sometimes I managed a decaf tea, which tasted terrible.

— ourselves to hydrate, hydrate — day and night — she with her pink 16-oz tumbler, me with the 12-oz blue —

Sipped sewage. Gulped sewage.

THE FIRST TIME I TOOK OFF THE DRESSINGS
AND ATTEMPTED A SHOWER I ENDED UP
FAINTING ON THE FLOOR OUTSIDE THE
BATHROOM.

Sour comical faces across the room as we attempted to sip together, massive quantities of lukewarm sewage to combat chemo constipation and to flush our respective poisons through our respective —

Pink Cup to the light to measure —

Blue Cup to the window (bitter laughter —

COMING TO OUT OF A CIRCULAR BLACKNESS,
JUST LIKE ON —

When the hearse glided through the traffic light on Hamlet Avenue it narrowly missed colliding with a car that failed to stop for our procession.

The hearse driver barked his horn.

$130 for the four digits, "within six weeks, weather permitting" —

Our driver muttered his disgust.

— not until she was safely in the —

    — CIRCULAR BLACKNESS, JUST LIKE ON —

    ▪ *... practical* things you can do now to live a long life that's as *good* and healthy and carefree —

How long she has been — he has been —

Elaborate network of —

— they have been —

We sighed a collective sigh, one last —

You, too — your turn —

                        — *right behind* —

What you do all day, reading *Martha* —

- ... *whether* you are 20 or 80, life can be meaningful, purposeful, and *beautiful* as long as you have the right guidance —

— gagged, gagged on well-meaning chocolate, powders, protein supplements —

- *Simplest Layer Cake Ever* (white buttercream with violets)

— exception of white pasta. Whole grain anything was inedible.

Sour toast.

Spicy anything was out. Spiced anything.

I dumped curried split pea soup down the sink. Ditto the Thai curry I'd made in advance, thinking, naively, I could stockpile —

Chocolate in all forms.

Coffee.

Thankfully I was able to eat hummus.

- ...*staying* active and healthy throughout your 'platinum' years —

— by far was water. Maybe our taste buds were not so much compromised as supercharged —

▪   ... you are in control of *how you live* every day —

We counted throughout the day and into the evening. I tried to encourage her.

— and what we recoiled from was the actual taste of municipally treated water, the cocktail of reservoir, sewage, petrochemicals, pharmaceuticals, animal runoff —

Three more!

It helped to use straws to gag down bigger sips.

Two more!

Lemon slices were recommended but equally —

Room temperature only.

Symmetry of *cotyledons* —

She was particularly susceptible to cold, including cold food. At the beginning I offered her a bite of ice cream I'd made, which caused her to scream as though she'd been stabbed in the jaw, scramble up from her rocker and spit with great violence all remaining traces in the sink.

Budding — blooming — some kind of violet perennials along the wall.

Pink rhododendrons —

Grass fills in one blade at a time.

Hopped up, nearsighted chipmunk scoots across the wall, down the steps and bangs up against the screen door.

— raised — ache — bloat —

Does she suspect I'm hoarding juicy nuts in the entry rather than half a bag of potting mix and a dirty push broom?

Clover creep and dandelions reclaim the scruffy —

— drip — leak — flutter —

Boxelders sunbathe, immobile, across the window screens.

— cough —

    BEST STRATEGY IS NOT TO —

— bump — twinge —

A small crew of men my parents hired many years ago leap out of a truck and proceed to leaf blast their way through the small back yard, small front yard, sucking up sticks and dandelions.

I intervene to inform them of my mother's death ten weeks ago. We muse about the prospect of eliminating Mr. W from the cemetery.

— any nonspecific — any —

That would be another company, says the leader.

Afterward, I discover numerous wintered over cigarette butts (walkers? drivers?) embedded in the front lawn along the sidewalk, though the small herb bed against the house is tidier, vacuumed of leaf debris.

Branches sway — birdhouses —

A package of Predascent© coyote-urine capsules in today's mail.

— pre-dawn *boo-wee* — *boo-wee* — *boo-wee* —

Orange tulips along the wall, and the cutest violet perennials, some of which have crept out onto the lawn in an arc, by invisible design.

'True' leaves on the *Serrano Tampiqueno!*

3:33 AM machination: (1) soak a Predascent© capsule (2) mash it up with the Jerry-curls in the Ziploc (3) dump the mock 'coyote' fur ball down the burrow —

"... bobcat urine has been shown to reduce woodchuck gnawing by 98% —"

My house, his house —

Biddle-biddle —

Predators*: coyotes, foxes, bobcats, raccoons, minks, black
bears, and weasels ...*

Searchlight moon.

Mapleshimmer.

Deterrents*: human hair, smelly socks, blood meal, bath soap,
liquid manure ...*

Birds in their nests. Peaceable (Suburban) Kingdom.

Literal scorched-earth yard. Too many drought
summers? Neglect?

More peat pot disintegration and pressure to transplant
outdoors, now the temperatures flirt with 60°, though
nothing as yet 'hardened off'.

Plush carpets *tsk-tsk* over fences and from across the
street.

Capsules to be scattered and watered "at 3½' intervals,
every four to five weeks".

Some of the hypergreen yards along the road bear
skullish flags jammed in the ground, *Pesticide Application.*

— 'all-natural' (the 'nature' of which is not made clear on the Patent Pending box, sporting a spooked woodchuck on hind legs —

— mini-Fenway parks, cemetery green —

Should one hold one's breath or —

Air through bald dry nostrils (clogged blood on tissue after tissue —

4:26 AM fantasy: tap the maple next spring, a *Martha*-proud project, enough to boil down to a single *Little House* tablespoon —

LOVE AND MEMORIES REMAIN

Lap number two — three —

SEE YOU IN HEAVEN

— that no one writes quaint verses on stones anymore.

Birch, azalea, lilacs curl around the graves.

Wide, looping lap —

The big Caterpillar sits idle over the weekend, having ripped open another field for development across the way, folding sod under and creating a large hill or a small mountain of earth to one side.

A (likely) veteran and his motorcycle make a quiet revolution.

— poison ivy? Rash or blotch directly beneath my scar.

Another veteran.

(The visiting nurse took one look —

Every day for two weeks I cleaned the dime-sized sore on her back, the biopsy site; spread a thin layer of Neosporin©; and covered it with a big square bandage. For some reason the site continued to ooze droplets of blood day after day.

For the briefest interval I went online to try and convince myself that the sore could be an abrasion from the johnny she wore at the —

LOVE AND MEMORIES

Mr. W's ancestors have long been partial to her daisies (ineffective wedding ring slammed against the upper window —

Red and green leaves —

Patch of eczema across the belly?

The terrycloth turbans <u>were</u> incredibly —

Red and yellow tulips along the wall perk as the morning progresses, petal peacocks —

Qu'est-ce que c'est all this reddened mulch in yard after yard? (Equivalent of Red Velvet cake?)

— clots and spikes —

A man paints his picket fence, spattering the sidewalk milky white.

— spotted with clots —

The morning of my biopsy results she vomited. I'd never before seen her once —

— *furred fontanel* —

I even imagined it was some sort of sympathetic stress response.

— right far neater than the —

Shadows across lawns.

Patch of eczema? — oval configuration just above the ribs—

Neosporin© across the dime-sized —

DON'T READ IF YOU'D RATHER SKIP THE GORY—

Seedlings strain for sunshine on the sills.

— left shoulder blade above the bra —

— IN MY MIND, YET STILL TRY TO IMAGINE --

The adorable purple flowers beside the daffodils are *Muscari* or 'grape hyacinths'.

— ONE MORE TRIP WEST BEFORE I SHUFFLE
OFF THIS MORTAL —

Bittersweet to see her perennials pop along the wall these past weeks.

RESCUE JUST TOOK HER AWAY.

A gift.

I'd never thought of gardens in that way.

Hot winds through the maple — buds rocking.

Harbinger —

I'M HEADING OUT.

Garden as legacy.

After one year, compulsory acclimation to the concave chest in the mirror; 'dog ear' bulges over the breast bone; pale pink scars (one neat, one flared) to the armpits. Some shirts fit better than —

Sweaters tend to camouflage —

BEST STRATEGY IS NOT TO —

— right armpit beneath my old scar. A thickening —

— one side, then the other —

Right under the scar! What were the odds?

— also stripes —

A definite —

Why not me —

— full body scan to 'stage' —

URINE DECREASE (tea-colored, concentrated)

The morning after my biopsy I got a haircut but said
nothing to the stylist, watching my head in the mirror
and the hair glance my shoulders on its way to the floor.

— tongue depressor scrape of cells —

I did wonder when I would need another — not for a
year (more than a year) —

The scan showed nothing but some irregularity in the left
knee, osteoarthritis that has plagued me for years.

— gradual forgetting, diminishment, as before, with —

She sent the sample away in an envelope via overnight courier to determine if I was —

This is inevitable.

(I was neither, despite mother — sister —

How this can —

— maternal great-aunts — possible grandmother —

Another sunrise, still and quiet.

SEE YOU IN HEAVEN

Much obliged.

How — how —

One revolution around Resurrection is approximately one half mile according to my odometer.

How —

Some days I can manage four, with effort. A year ago I did six or seven routinely.

    "— can have a toxic effect on the heart —"

— *sleep, sleep that knits up the ravell'd sleave of —*

"— tested for heart problems before starting and continuously monitored for developing —"

Waiting on the lilacs.

Bunches in clear vases. Our whiffleballs sailed in the branches, necessitating tricky rescues.

Executive decision: I have fired the lawn care company (six years of noise, battering into submission all living —

Waiting —

Noise pollution — battalion —

I purchase an electric lawn mower online, reasonably confident I can maneuver this across the crumbly brown yard for exercise, variation on walking. I am not, after all, an invalid.

Not —

      Maybe —

The *Boston Pickling cotyledons* yellow and shrivel, near dropping —

I read that even a petite woman can push this machine around 'like a vacuum cleaner'.

2:24 AM reverie: replace the brown front lawn with a lovely, climate-zone appropriate, drought-tolerant Wildflower Meadow ...

'True' *Genovese Italian* basil leaves — miniature ruffled, doll-sized —

The blotch beneath my scar holds steady and if anything, appears to have —

Two small insect bites?

— day after day of real spring, the first in recent —

Waiting for the soil to warm before 'hardening' the transplants.

Maple buds, russet-hued —

One more week?

Mr. W suns himself on the cemetery —

— my oatmeal-wheat-flax bread invention —

Puppet? Stuffed animal?

A single revolution, or one half mile, seems well beyond—

Like something on a children's show, shuffling down the wall.

Three mountains of soil and sod in the clearing,
awaiting—

LOVE AND MEMORIES

Mesclun thicket thrives in the freestanding window box.

This is a wonderful gift to your loved one.

I waltz the box from sunny spot to sunny spot, sunporch
to living room and back to cool sunporch for the night.

Near daily hyperventilation: *incredible* findings with
exciting genetic implications. White-coated spokespeople
expressing guarded enthusiasm, though the news itself is
consistently —

— SHIFT AT THE HOUSE OF HORRORS —

— *worst* breast cancers now linked with the *worst*
leukemias linked with the *worst* endometrial *blah blah* —

SAID HE SUSPECTED IMMEDIATELY FROM CT—

— but they've been <u>linked</u>!

Wisp-blue sunshine. Dandelions proliferate across the
chewed, sorry yard.

Front lawn as Wildflower —

Where to transplant all these *Boston Pickling* cukes.

She mailed me packets of wildflower seeds some months ago; dilemma of —

— new or redundant bills from a chemo appointment eleven months (?) ago. I can't quite figure out if they are legit or not, or whether they're just now catching up —

(At the hardware store, I eye the canning accoutrements lunatically, shelves of shiny Mason jars.)

Two sets of cancer bills, mine and hers.

I keep the substantial, growing stacks on separate sides of the room to maintain some —

> WENT 'VERY WELL'. TOOK OUT THE TUMOR
> AND—

— a dozen of these idiotic bills, one for every single —

I would like a big bowl of popcorn and many hours of nothing but —

— oatmeal-wheat-flax toast *extraordinaire* —

Maybe five hours sleep.

Pernicious — nightly —

I laid down my head —

Maybe four hours.

One year out, six months post-rads, an almost normal
feeling to the area below the armpit and along the scar
though the armpit itself, from which sprout a few slow-
growing wiry hairs, remains insensate.

What to do with a multitude of *Serrano Tampiqueno* and
Santa Fe peppers, should they produce well?

I have eschewed deodorant for over a year.

Discovery: <u>pickle</u> peppers in white vinegar with a pinch
of sugar and serve over garlic lo mein.

I smell better. Neutral.

Plant the hot pepper seedlings along the heat-retaining
wall in the back yard.

Prune back some daisies —

 The red ones are tulips, too, with 'double petals' — so, so
lovely —

— and hope that Mr. W is not partial to spicy —

For a change I walk up to Spring Water Drive, a few
blocks from the house at the top of the modestly steep
Oregon Avenue.

GETTING READY TO GO TO HER 'GYM'.

Stroller's pace past small, aging ranch houses until the
top of the hill where the road smoothes, the properties
expand, the grass greens, and a cul-de-sac emerges,
manicured lawns with hints of pools in the distance, and
long tree-cloaked driveways.

WORKING ON UPPER ARM STRENGTH, SOME
STAIRS, SHOE TYING, ETC.

How many, how many times they can friggin' charge —

SUBJECT: HIGHLY UNPLEASANT NEWS

Today's paper describes yesterday's fire on Spring Water,
at the Yippy Dog house where I discovered the road
blocked off, two idling fire engines and a tv cameraman
in his car at the top of the hill.

— succession of 'amended' chemotherapy bills from a
year ago, each one with its own nauseating co-pay of —

"... gave Buddy oxygen at the scene. He later died."

My bills, not *hers* —

"The third family Yorker, Chewy, died —"

Pair of slippers, spinach, fresh strawberries at the farm
stand is exertion for the day.

Blue Cross vs. Medicare — hers the more labyrinthine,
particularly with layers of supplemental —

I prune the rosemary in the herb bed, browned sprigs trying to rebound from winter, with a series of satisfying snips.

Byzantine billing practices — primitive typed sheets, *sans* return envelope.

Tough weeds ('saplings', not poison ivy, I am apprised), tough roots ripping through the earth.

Difficult, if not impossible, to determine what, where, whom, why —

May sun so strong I must retreat for a few hours.

Maple buds redden, overtaking the gold —

Lilac buds —

Butter block forsythia —

Too exhausted to drive the mile to Resurrection, I walk the main road again, turn up at Oregon and lurch along in slow motion. When the modest incline makes my heart pound —

     "— toxic effect —"

The doomed pair barked themselves into tizzies whenever I was fifty yards away.

I turn back.

Were they smelling me from afar? (No deodorant.)

Podcasts seeping through my earbuds?

Tizzy, tizzy of barking —

Last summer one of the Yippys broke through his invisible electric fence and charged, barking with all the ferocity he could muster. All I could do was stumble across the street and up onto a neighbor's showcase lawn, envisioning teeth in my calf, subsequent infection, hospitalization and death, lacking, for all intents and purposes, any immune system.

"The fireman gave him oxygen."

Tizzy, tizzy (Toto-esque, though, so cute!) up against my sneaker.

I waved my arm: "Go home!"

BODY TEMPERATURE (increasingly cool to the —

Magically, he turned and fled.

I lurch-hurried as best I could down the hill as I heard him charging again — tizzy, tizzy — paws tap-tapping on the concrete road.

Was that *Chewy*? *Buddy*?

We started the day before she died.

— or the one that survived — *Marley?*

The machine made a racket, as it did with my sister, and my father.

NB: Coma + Oxygen = Impending —

— seasonal flowers; uber-green grass; rotating themed mailboxes on the cusp of the dreamy cul-de-sac.

RESTLESSNESS (repetitive motions —

(My father did last almost a week, refusing to Go Gently into That Good —

I tried to remove the apparatus but the tubing got stuck around her head. My aunt stepped in. I switched off the gravelly, humming machine.

Buddy? Chewy? Marley?

I laid my head down —

Red buds overtake the gold.

Lilac progress —

Four revolutions at Resurrection. Using the wind, sail-like, to blow me around —

I switched off the machine.

No year. Dirt pale, baked, crumbly with one or two footprints.

— obligatory flag, the veteran of the four.

(Who is walking on the grave?)

We buried him — closed casket — in a polo shirt and sweatpants.

Sunken; settled down below grass level.

— blue nightgown, purchased under duress, three days prior, by loved ones dispatched on this errand. Someone cut the back with a pair of scissors to approximate a hospital johnny. They'd bought a blue one and a matching pink —

My mother carried this outfit to the funeral home, passing the bag across the desk to the associate, who put it on the floor out of sight.

Mémère: her nice fuchsia dress, I believe.

Pépère: his best suit, for certain, last of the open casket era.

QUITE A BIT OF SWELLING IN HER —

How the well dressed elders must look upon their
children, dressed indifferently by *their* children, a
generation inclined to cremation though cremated bodies,
too, must be attired.

— ANTIBIOTICS —

Fresh flowers replace plastic in marker vases beside the
graves.

Carnations, geraniums, roses, tulips, lilies —

RESCHEDULE CT SCAN THAT WAS DUE LAST —

White azaleas — pink azaleas among —

... HER SECOND INFUSION AND THEY'RE HAVING
TROUBLE WITH THE PORT, AND SHE HAS TO
GET AN X-RAY —

Or, as Kate Hepburn says, a "bow-ah" —

— AND IT IS 'KINKED UP AND TWISTED',
UNUSABLE, SO SHE HAS TO HAVE IT REMOVED
AND A SECOND PORT PUT IN —

Pull up the old flavorless oregano, the large bush which
survived prodigious winter snows (as did the thyme and
rosemary), and replace with the Greek oregano seedlings,
modest leaf growth in two peat pots thus far.

— AHEAD OF ME BY ONE INFUSION.

As I begin to tackle the green mound with the hand rake
(?), a dirt clump moves.

I ignore the moving dirt clump, imagining it to be a shifting as a result of my assiduous scraping, but the clump moves again and a muddy head rises up.

Baby, hairless chipmunk?

Upon closer inspection, Muddy Clumphead exhibits a rhythmic throb, clamoring, yet failing, to bury himself again.

WE LIKE TO KEEP SCORE.

To the best of my fauna faculties, I classify *frog* or *toad*, and vacate the mound of insipid oregano for another day.

Frogs as 'excellent' friends of gardens, eating many 'bad' insects —

The faux poison ivy-sapling comes up easily. Other woody, thready roots snap off, indignant.

Much soil is quite terrible — rocky and rooty — yet herbs flourish and toads reproduce; snows have come and gone with no ill effects.

Already the butter forsythia begins to green, straddling two seasons.

Thirties in the morning and the furnace kicking in. Sunshine in the afternoon with windows flung open, flirting with 70°.

Sleep with windows open and wake to a chill.

I lay aside, but do not pack away, my thermal pjs.

Put it on; take it off —

('Lasagna' pipedream abandoned, beyond my finite —

Mail dread.

The Honda she drove to the market, to church, the mall, the senior center to play cards clicks and flutters, refusing to turn over, three months since the funeral. A neighbor says *start it every so often* so I do, revving the motor gently, once a week or so, but still the battery dies.

My bills, her bills ...

A burly dude takes a flat blue gadget from his truck, attaches some cables — defibrillates —

— beating heart —

In ten months I've racked up over $330,000 in gross charges:

- Biopsy.

- Two breasts.

- Failed port insertion leading to a partially collapsed lung.

- Successful port insertion.

- Successful port removal.

- Eight dose-dense chemo infusions.

- Scans; labwork; many quarts of blood drawn.

- Eight immunity booster Neulasta© horse shots at __? apiece.

- Thirty-three radiation zappings.

- Many appointments and follow-ups of the eight-minute variety, each of which were and are billed to insurance at —

Her Medicare: $25,000 full reimbursement for *each* of her twelve —

— **pupils enlarged, eyes fixed on a certain spot —**

— finite heartbeats (could we see — we could not —

... chemotherapy alone, not counting doctors; hospital stays; visits to the ER; the broken foot; colon resection; hip replacement; four ambulance trips; rehabilitation;

nursing home; visiting nurses; equipment; transport; hospice —

Half million?

Delusional *rah rah.*

Million?

Blah blah <u>statistics</u> *blah blah blah* <u>outcome</u> —

Ten months —

Blah blah <u>very good</u> *blah blah* —

Co-pay. Co-pay. Knocking on her grave —

Knocking on my —

If only we could —

— even <u>with</u> her secondary and supplemental insurances—

All hope abandon, ye who enter —

She could not, with the neuropathy, hold a fork, a pen, a cup —

I take the beige Honda on the highway to recharge the battery. The car is quite peppy, grateful to be out in the fresh air.

All hope —

Beneath the hood, a few dried leaves leftover from last autumn, when she was still behind the wheel.

Sets of bills, duplicates, mistakes, lame bills without envelopes or clear addressee, bills for 'miscellaneous hospital charges' — WTF? (my bills clearer than hers, my clinic of higher —

She spent her last years as a widow buried in bills and bureaucracy —

> *TWO* DUELING CANCER TREATMENT PLANS, LIKE PUTTING ON THE MOST COMPLICATED AND UGLY (FILL IN THE NAUSEATING EVENT OF YOUR CHOICE) —

Fatigue — fatigue — *clickety-click* —

> "... study of cancer patients in the *Annals of Internal Medicine* found that many doctors didn't quite tell patients the truth about their prognosis. "

— scroll, scroll – fugue — scroll —

> SORRY FOR THE DELAY BUT I'VE BEEN DEALING WITH CRISIS #2, MORE CANCER. YES, MY MOTHER THIS TIME (AGAIN),

> "Doctors were up front about their patients' estimated survival 37% of the time; refused to give

an estimate 23% of the time; and told patients something else 40% of the time."

YES, A FRESH KIND NOT PREVIOUSLY SEEN IN OUR EXTENSIVE —

Cool, dewy, clover-dripping dawn.

"Around 70% of the discrepant estimates were overly optimistic."

Good day to strategize how and where to move seedlings from temperate, sheltered windowsills to yard of scary elements.

Mr. W astride his hole, vigilant.

Sunday, Mother's Day.

Newborns in the burrow? Mommy W? Scritch-scratching through Union soldier bones?

HAD TO CALL 911 —

The first.

Stomach blotch faded almost —

Daffodils done for.

The dead bell

Last gasp for tulips, though the lilacs are starting to show.

Rhododendrons shedding petals.

Mr. W creeps out in the morning to keep the dandelion population down.

                                        Somebody's done for

Russet maple filling in.

                                        Somebody's —

Waiting on the year —

Boo-wee — boo-wee — boo-wee —

Clipped chives, three great bushes along the wall, one flowering purple puffballs.

Boo-wee — boo-wee —

Half an hour in the garden-to-be, one strip along the fence where I grew peppers and cucumbers as a girl.

No spade to be found in the long purged garage, but a rusty pitchfork in the shed.

Ground mangled with ropy pointless roots.

I jam the fork down and bend with my full weight, terrified that Rusty will snap off the handle and impale me. Palm-sized boulders are the current crop.

— peppers, tomatoes, cucumbers —

Every so often the most satisfying splitting noise, like comical pant seams, breaking up root masses in blessed whole chunks.

NO MORE COFFEE FOR ME.

Lilacs mock from their vantage atop the wall.

BREADY PRODUCTS SEEM PARTICULARLY AWFUL. SOME THINGS FINE, LIKE PASTA WITH TOMATO SAUCE AND SALAD WITH OIL AND VINEGAR DRESSING.

The strong spring sun curtails my best intentions.

SOMETHING ACIDIC?

Muscari holding their own.

FIRST DAY I CAN HOLD MYSELF UP AND NOT CREEP AROUND THE HOUSE LIKE —

Around 9:00 AM Mr. W sidles along the wall, flattens himself beneath the chain-link fence and into the neighbor's yard to graze plusher grass, with a side of birdseed scattered beneath two feeders.

— vague recollection of determined, prepubescent self, dousing tomatoes with the hose, channeling Pa, Ma and Laura —

Weeding on hands and knees on the folded, repurposed blue bathmat.

— strong sun — glare —

Tear-glue from my tear ducts sealed the lids overnight so they were difficult to crust open in the morning.

During the day I kept a wet hand towel nearby to cope with gluey secretions.

Every fifteen minutes I shuffled to the bathroom to bathe the sticky glue from my eyes.

Lids stuck, attempts to pry them open with superstrong blinks.

> NEUTROPENIC, EVEN WITH THE SHOT, AND
> SLIGHTLY —

Gluey vision (eyedrops useless), long given up on contacts —

> MISPLACED MY GLASSES, A NEVER IN MY
> LIFETIME OCCURRENCE, WHICH WOUND UP ON
> THE FLOOR.

Tear-glue as chemo residue?

> THE OTHER DAY I WAS ABOUT TO LEAVE FOR
> MY APPOINTMENT IN MY SLIPPERS.

My onc flummoxed. The optical glue factory went on for a few weeks.

Every day lashes floated in my eyes and fell out of my head.

THIS MORNING MY MOTHER LOST HER CLOTH
GROCERY BAGS AT THE —

Lashes beneath the lids —

How lilacs know it's Mother's Day —

— jabbing — poking — stabbing my corneas. Tops and bottoms.

I have known the ineffable cuteness of buttercups, hundreds dotting the backyard, just as the forsythia starts to shed along the driveway, picking up the yellow slack.

Every year!

Without access to a spade I am limited to the hand spade, or is this called 'trowel', inquired the dunce.   Maybe all I can manage —

Showers, showers predicted at long —

— voluminous discharge, too, quarts and quarts of viscous snot (fattest maxis useless) —

Impossible to lift and hold lashless lids to move contacts in or —

I blotted the snot, scraping as much off the pad stack as I could with toilet paper, every half hour, for —

Boo-wee —

I sat and stood and trudged down the sidewalk and sprawled on the couch and slept in the de facto wet diaper for days, weeks —

Boo-wee — boo-wee — boo-wee —

— pried open for a juicy clip of tissue (ultrasound <u>negative</u> —

Mr. W inhales some greenery beside the neighbor's raised flower bed.

Cardinal watches on the ground nearby — *oh, the Cardinal and the Woodchuck should be* —

I wailed so loudly the waiting room must have been traumatized.

Boo-wee — boo-wee — boo-wee gunfire (maple choir—

— the mercy of Mr. W; menagerie of birds; squirrels; chipmunks; Tan Bunny; insects; mildew; disease; soil bacteria; blight and —

Overnight transformation, every inch of branch flush with wine-colored leaves, cooling shade for the next five—

Biddle-biddle —

To keep them inside, safe, irrationally so (more roots
poke through the deteriorating peat boxes) —

Thatchy (squirrel?) nest at the very top obscured now
until October.

Predator principle.

Lilacs — for a stop-motion camera —

> PASTA OKAY, SO ARE SALSA, SALAD,
> AVOCADOS, REFRIED BEANS ...

— baby shower across the brown baked yard. Tease of
drops — drought —

Darwinian advantage to the buttercup?

Good to have a break from the sun. Too much sun —

Come, come and eat me.

> WHAT A GEM OF A BOOK! MADE ME SO
> *HOMESICK* FOR A TIME AND PLACE THAT CAN
> NEVER BE —

Battle or ambush?

> — SINCE I'VE TAKEN SUCH PLEASURE IN ANY
> BOOK. HAPPY TO SNUGGLE WITH IT IN THE
> SHADE OF THE MAPLE.

... gnarly soil; pecking sparrows; typhoon winds;
downbursts; insect gangs; unfiltered sky —

> TOO WEAK, STILL ON LIQUID DIET (RAZOR
> BLADES ON THE SIDE OF MY TONGUE) THOUGH
> TODAY I CAN MOVE MY TONGUE WITHOUT
> SHOOTING, BLINDING —

Intermittent downbursts wash the walkway in the yard,
the butt-specked sidewalk in front of the house.

Cleansing.

Baked brown yard darkens; matted brown weeds suck
greedily.

Dandelions leap to attention as Mr. W tiptoes the wall.

Fresh smells —

An hour passes. I forget the kingdom I inhabit.

> NONE OF THIS IS FUN.

Dandelions loom after the rains.

I remember (blotch on trunk faded to almost —

> — A COUPLE OF POSSIBLE INFECTIONS AND
> DISCOVERED TO HAVE —

— removed within hours, as the snow started: hospital
bed; nightstand table; reclining lift chair (never used);

portable commode (used twice with so much torturous assistance she may have half-willed herself to die, which she did, forty-eight hours later); oxygen machine; pair of oxygen tanks —

Chives skyward, several inches overnight.

    —"person to person by the contaminated hands of caregivers" —

Lilacs fill and fade to pink.

The hospice nurse retrieved the morphine. We agreed she departed *just in time* before the blizzard —

Cotyledons yellow and curled.

I pinch some off, wary of this transgression.

— explosive snot-gush as soon as I rolled out of bed — stood — all day — days —

Might come in handy. (She didn't grasp my aside, and how could she?)

The entry screen windows are covered top to bottom with strange Winged Insects.

Frantic search online: harmless flying ants vs. foundation-chomping termites?

Termites come out in spring after 'heavy rains'.

— broom, broom them out the —

— wet, wet diaper —

Open the screen to let them out (not budging) —

Some seem to be ants.

Some def have 'wings'?

— assured by vague sources that they "will not bite"?

Within the hour they do disappear, gone up perhaps, in a termite vapor, not unlike the memorable 'glittering cloud' episode in *On the Banks of Plum Creek.*

Cukes and zukes appear to flower when I turn my head for a couple of hours. Even the hydroponics.

Transplant ASAP, you procrastinator —

Cool showers. Bits of sun.

Maybe too late? 'Root-bound'?

Plan: Wednesday, the beginning of a moderate stretch, to plunk things in —

Dandelions bend after the rains.

Weedy shoots dot the yard beside the front steps and the rhododendron (azalea?) bushes, astonishing rose blooms.

Taxes — Banking — House —

Lilacs take their Mother's Day cue, pops of perfume on
brisk breezes, though clustered high beyond my grasp.

— Honda — Medicare file folders in the massive desk —

Butter block forsythia showers the driveway, bush gone
green —

Gene Kelly sailorish, red and white —

My father's records, too, his own cancer narrative printed
neatly, stapled in a separate file folder (harder to
summon now, three, three and a half years —

Hundreds of recipe index cards in her distinct Catholic
penmanship —

Horizontal stripes *do* —

— file folder labeled —

Flour and sugar tins are fifty, sixty years old?

Rubber-banded, alphabetized packs in two wooden
boxes: *Cakes and pies. Miscellaneous desserts. Main courses.*

A year (?): tidy small finances; cull old boxes in
basement—

Swedish Apple; Apricot; Blueberry; Blueberry Cranberry;
Boston Creme; Coconut Cream ...

"*very 'cute' senior*"

(concomitant Bartleby malaise) —

"*sweet little gal*"

Bedside bureau drawer, class of 1950 —

"*ardent baseball fan*" "*swell girl*"
"*hardworking business pupil*"

Boxes and boxes and spider webs. Creaky rusted filing
cabinet —

"*nicest blue eyes I ever saw*"

... Lemon-Lime Chiffon; Lemon Meringue; Mincemeat Walnut;
Peach with Almond Nut Topping; Pineapple Cream; Pumpkin
with Ginger Streusel ...

"*Have fun at commencement.*"

... Raisin Nut; Strawberry Rhubarb; Strawberry Yogurt; Sweet
Potato; Tangerine Chiffon ...

White plastic blueberry buckets on the basement wall
(roped around our necks —

"*Don't come home with the milkman.*"

Bureau top drawer: the 'Reacher', pinching pole hand-extension that allowed her to retrieve slippers or the paper post-hip fracture.

Long yellow shoehorn on steroids. She (we) pushed her swollen feet into slippers, then graduated to sneakers (such a milestone!) —

 Round yellow sponge on a stick to 'wash feet'. Did she ever —

Contraption to tie and untie laces?

Personal hygiene foam (package of adult diapers —

The dying person might experience varied and mixed —

Kerfuffle of trying to hire a contractor to install grab bars in the shower — one vertical, one horizontal — though she would only take two more —

(They did say *squamous or basal cell* —

> — NOT IN HER ARM, AS SUGGESTED, BUT IN THE SAME PLACE, THREADED OUTSIDE THE CLAVICLE INSTEAD OF UNDERNEATH, BUT IN THE 'SAME' POCKET.

The lesion biopsy site never seemed to heal, oozing drops of blood every time I removed the big square bandage.

> JUST TO TORTURE US FURTHER, THE SURGEON CALLED AT 5:30 LAST NIGHT TO TELL HER OF THESE NEW PLANS.

We were told this was —

— terrific shriek —

SHE WILL TRY OUT HER SHINY NEW PORT TOMORROW AND REPORT.

I raised her to a sitting, but no —

— siren — sirens —

P.S. WE DON'T EVER WANT TO THINK ABOUT PORTS AGAIN.

How much sap from this lone maple — <u>next</u> spring —

— sirens —

Plastic bag of plastic gloves —

I laundered the new blue cotton twin blanket.   Also the set of new white twin —

— single sheet of my father's entitled *Various symptoms:* "*waning appetite ... general weakness ... breathless for mild activity ...* "

Plastic bag of disposable eyedroppers (<u>tongue</u>, not eyes—

"... paleness ... sleep soundly but wake up tired ...
cold hands ..."

— new twin bed with new bedding; wheelchair; hospital
bed with new bedding —

USE 4 DROPS SUBLINGUALLY EVERY 4
HOURS

— set of email pages disseminating updates to the family:
"The doctors seem to think it is lymphoma. Because of the
involvement of the meninges (brain area) treatment would be
more —"

Rolled up and rolled down compression stockings (her
feet were blocks of ice in my –

"The man in the next bed is some windbag who they both
know, who M used to hide from in the grocery store because he
talked so much. We are trying to ignore him without actual
rudeness —"

Chill winds make a comeback, though lilacs bloom high,
well out of my —

Flyer invitation celebrating 'survivorship'.

Crisp yellow flowers on the earlier *Boston Picklings; Black*
Beauty zukes not far behind.

Bad sign? Premature fertility?

I tear in half and jam the pieces into the recycling bag.

Root-bound?

Hands, too. I rubbed them between mine.

I thought I had more time.

Raised to a sitting, but no —

Bald; anemic; neutropenic; dehydrated; light-headed;
stirrups and 'juicy clip' (much later I read that painkillers
are strongly advised before this —

Frost advisory?!

— dozen bagels with the same oatmeal-flax-dough,
packing the freezer ahead of more company.

Waiting on the year —

Hair in the usual places, though sparser.

— slow lashes, slowest —

Glory of peeing <u>straight</u> —

(Also my sister's newspaper column saved on the
computer, thanking my parents for their support after *her*
surgery —

Boxes of tampons, diaper-maxis, thin maxis, minis?
(farewell, farewell —

You're a wonderful daughter —

— mother —

— siren — sirens —

Reproductive stress? Root-bound?

Mr. W missing in action? Or in the burrow — birthing pups?

Tired, tired, sore, as though beaten with a club, after deigning to tackle the small but challenging lawn with the new mower and the 100' neon orange extension cord picked up at the hardware store.

The flying ant-mites have decamped without a —

Up — down — around — beneath — across big patches of mostly dirt flecked with dandelions; up and down three sets of yard 'stairs' on three levels.

Rake-scraped the front strip near the sidewalk, the Butt Festival sprinkled with junk-food wrappers; gathered the littered dirt in a basket; left the dried clump of somebody's dog shit present for another —

— stars — briefly (what was I thinking?)

On the other side of the bush facing away from the house, dozens of lilacs —catching more sun?

I clip enough for two big vases.

My neighbor K— greets me over the fence and says lilacs are her favorites, too, like my mother, with whom she shared a birthday. That they put the St. Bernard down (bone cancer) six weeks ago.

— muscle — *mowing* — memory —

That the garage squirrels are driving her crazy, that mothballs haven't helped, that our resident 'chuck has been prowling under their cars, that she can't mow the cemetery border because of the poison ivy —

As advertised, the mower is easy to operate —

That of course they'll keep an eye on the house while I'm away.

So gray and cold, I put the heat on.

That she misses her, too.

— even for a small woman —

(Thursday could be 80°.)

New container babies: *Slo-Bolt Cilantro* in the wide basket emerges as wiry stalks, several inches all at once.

Ditto *Giant of Italy* parsley in the blue ceramic pot.

I laid my head on her —

— prophylactic mastectomies (*something* as better than —

Sudden invasion of SuperAnts on my desk, bedspread, curtains — thinking it's winter again?

He, too, used the lightweight wheelchair for a brief time, but was moved to a hospice facility before the need for a commode.

— be spirited away in a (Bartleby) matter of — *healthcare proxy — beneficiaries —*

— shocking white and sparse (lesions had broken through on her scalp, on her 54-year-old mastectomy scar—

— *living* —

He palpated abdomen and liver —

I laid my head on her chest —

I'm right behind you.

Sun breaks — winds — fat robins peck the newly shorn—

Maybe it won't happen to —

—'eco-burials' with bamboo caskets (cremation debatably more —

Yank up the insipid oregano.

Plant the *Serrano* and the *Santa Fe* chiles against the wall.

Transplant basil seedlings.

I do use jars to trap and set free errant ladybugs, boxelders, *Charlotte's Web* spiders in the house but these inch-long ants have got to —

Direct-seed more cilantro and parsley.

Prune leggy thyme.

Folds of paper towel — light (no remorse) crackles.

After a couple of hours in the yard I am creaky-kneed; winded; off-balance as I squat and rise from the old blue bathmat.

Another Mutant Ant slithers across the beige —

Hack, hack through the soil with her ancient implements, a scoopy trowel with teeth; the hand scraping thing; the sticky pruning shears.

Shape the rosemary plant, which has rebounded after the snowy winter, flush with green needles.

Another Mutant slithers —

Cut back the fragrant thyme which has flung branches willy-nilly across the plot.

Another Mutant —

Revisit the mound of insipid 'golden' oregano with the rusty pitchfork (pray the muddy 'E.T.' frog has vacated); lift up and beneath; rip roots.

The clump comes up neat and whole.

Toss the golden clump across the walk, beneath the maple in the shade in a dusty, grassless patch.

Another Mutant —

Pitchfork a new foot-wide strip of sod along the walkway beside the mailbox, connecting stairs with herb plot.

This endeavor proves to be a major undertaking, not the least of which is the transport of six renegade, lichen-stained concrete bricks from the wall beneath the lilacs.

These orphan bricks are about a foot long and weigh at least twenty? pounds apiece.

Pray not to drop the damn things on my toes in the ten-yard or so journey from wall to plot.

Sun peek-a-boos as the maple sashays —

Scoopy trowel a hollow for each brick, careful to avoid wounding any of several stretchy worms which writhe up and out of the fresh —

Worms are *not frogs* —

 Sore, sore, long dormant leg muscles. Skullcap tightness around my —

Winter (furnace this morning); spring (cool, cool breezes); summer (tomorrow, 80°) —

Waiting, waiting on the year —

Harden these seedlings.

Cannot keep my eyes —

That *she went so fast.*

I nod and look away into my bouquet of sun-baked lilacs.

"This completes the arrangement."

She'd brought over the emergency bed pan and held her upright while I wiped; maneuvered her back into the hospital bed; showed us how to position her head close to the wall with the sheet beneath the near dead weight—

I carried remembrance cards, the nice laminated ones, up the street to these stalwart neighbors —

— *goodbye*, unknowing, for the last —

— a half century of shared —

Biddle-biddle quank-quank heralds the coming summer, symphonic waves from the old —

Skull cap sensation —

Then nothing.

— *boo-wee* — *boo-wee* —

As the cemetery fills in, a thicket of leaves obscures the opening to Mr. W's burrow.

— secret bird scale —

— bomb ticking inside a suitcase. I climbed on a chair in a classroom to get everyone's attention. I turned seniors (elderly) away at the door. They didn't understand. I grappled with a laptop to retrieve the precise time of detonation, though a calm throughout the room, my singular knowledge —

Fat robins peck the freshly turned —

— before the dénouement —

peace and comfort

Mr. W cruises clover —

spirit and heart

Harden the seedlings —

Hot winds and sun —

Peat pots of basil, zukes, cukes on the plastic tray, the
cardboard —

"Last night I dreamed I went to —

— earthworm in the cakey, chocolate dirt —

— gradual, so as not to windburn; sunburn —

Growling mower —

Dawn's early *biddle-biddle-biddle* —

Outside the bathroom window, Mr. W fraternizes in the
cemetery with two fresh 'pups', lolling on rocks.

Boo-wee — boo-wee — quank-quank — quank-quank —

**The most appropriate interventions at this stage are comfort-
enhancing —**

Make that <u>three</u> —

Alleged lifecycle: (1) sleep (2) scamper out for clover
buffet, hypervigilant (nose a-twitching) (3) sun on rocks
(4) scamper home (5) disappear down burrow hole

(6) sleep (7) scamper out for clover —

Truncal muscles and thighs; calves mooing (surfeit of pitchfork activity, ripping mystery roots down to China (?), three foot long cords —

Biddle-biddle —

(I did try to lift the tubes from around her —

I decide to abridge the full hardening, as seedlings 'appear' hardy enough (am I fool?), having long outgrown the peat boxes and begun to flower yellow.

Temps look moderate for the foreseeable future.

"... grab bars and hand rails to fit every need —"

Happier buried in earth.

Many hours of preparation, root ripping along the fence beneath the lilacs.

Hacking through the mass of chives along the wall to make room —

> *Bench; tub transfer kit (300 lbs.); ADL hip kit; grab bar, 18": $189.79; Walker, Youth Guardian 30 Wheels; Install (2) grab bars, LABOR: $65.00; O$_2$ 2-liter*

— snip of mesclun from the prolific sunporch window box, tangled onto my sandwich —

> *Bed – Hi-Lo Electric, Comfort Therapeutic Mattress, Commode — Bedside Over Bed Table, Wheelchair —*

Dust-dry dirt, though perennials manage — the 'fittest'—

> <u>*Interventions*</u>*: Transfer (bed to chair); Shower; Hair Care; Mouth Care; Make Bed; Skin Care; Sponge Bath; Dress Pt; Toileting; Emotional Support (EACH VISIT)*

At last, two neat rows of *Boston Pickling* cukes and *Black Beauty* zuke plants; two rows of *Genovese* basil —

PHYSICAL SIGNS: an orderly progression of physical changes

— a *Serrano Tampiqueno* and a *Santa Fe* pepper plant —

Caron calls to follow up —

— the *Dwarf Siberian* kale, the *Giant of Italy* parsley and direct-seeded *Slo-Bolt* cilantro —

Recognizing Signs & Symptoms

> <u>*ICD9*</u>*: 174.9 Malign Neopl Breast NOS (Primary)*
> <u>*ICD9*</u>*: 197.0 Secondary Malig Neo Lung*

The plastic comfort bracelet insured no 'extraordinary measures'.

> *ICD9*: *197.7 Secondary Malig Neo Liver*
> *ICD9*: *198.2 Secondary Malig Neo Skin*

SPIRITUAL AND EMOTIONAL

Mr. W was 'Ms.' W all along?

> *Morphine Sulfate (concentrate) by mouth solution 20 mg/ml*

— children ('pups'?) on the sun-baked rock. Rapacious newborns learning to chomp all greenery in sight.

BODY TEMPERATURE (increasingly cool to –

Keep the poison ivy pruned?

> *Maybe it won't —*

They might be Disney —

Poison ivy curls over the wall.

Clang of pitchfork on rock produces the desired effect — skitterish scampering down the woodchuck hole for their afternoon tea.

After removing some of the longer branches (a stubborn one whips me across the face) to make the burrow opening less hospitable, I rinse pitchfork and gloves with the hose, then shower to try and minimize any —

— affirm the individual's ongoing value to you —

All seedlings in the ground in a burst of effort — bending and creaking — hacking and scraping — scooping and pressing, careful not to deluge my darlings with the stream of —

— good you will carry forward —

Basil astride the spent tulips.

Peppers sheltered against the purple flowering chives.

Scatter of carrot seed beside the withered daffodils.

Beneath the lilac, cukes and zukes brave the winds.

Robins dart in and out of the rows, worm-drunk.

JUNE

*"It is only when I stand painting before my easel
that I feel in any way alive."*

VINCENT VAN GOGH, LETTERS

Soil in hand, broken apart, dust-cloud —

(That tool is called a 'cultivator'.)

Brave, brave, heads bend to the puddle-logged —

Shivering, waiting on the sun —

Where I plugged the chipmunk hole by the maple, a
mushroom cap has emerged the size of a baseball.

— stenciled in: *2013*

**— shallow breaths with periods of no breathing (5 to 30
seconds and up to a full —**

Grasses filling out the plot.

Azaleas shedding.

The big lot across the path plowed bare, ready for seeding.

Hold your loved one's hand.

Mother and daughter creep among the new and the old—

Awash in lilacs — zephyr —

Clouds muscle in —

What to do with the rotting cilantro in the crisper drawer. I flip the reeking, browning bunch toward the burrow hole like a ring-toss.

Newborns circle, wary.

Speak gently.

If only the stench might overtake, encourage an exodus—

> WE DO RALLY AROUND ONE ANOTHER, EVEN
> THE PAIRINGS WHO DON'T ORDINARILY —

Counted <u>four</u> this morning, two of which appeared to be engaged in suspiciously procreative activity.

> ... ANY FEAR OR EVEN APPREHENSION...

Seedlings holding their own beneath the lilacs; among the perennials along the wall; in the small curved herb plot against the house.

Gloved fingers: greeny glow-worm arches her back; long brown earthworm plays (or *is*) dead.

Unmolested in their first days, embracing the gentle shower overnight, the much abated winds.

Monarch floats among the spent daffodils.

Bees nudge the edges of my pitchfork.

Fat robins rejoice at the tilled earth.

Five new buds on her orchid.

Your loved one may seem unresponsive, withdrawn, or in a comatose-like —

Christmas cacti dormant.

Death of the African violet.

Dust bombs between thumb and forefinger —

This indicates preparation for release, a detaching from surroundings and relationships, and a beginning —

Yard sponge, treading over moss, sneakers sinking in the soft ground. Chocolate clay and compost along the wall.

NOTHING NEW EXCEPT CREEPING AROUND,
TRYING TO DEAL WITH OTHER ISSUES THIS
WEEK WHICH ARE JUST TOO —

Specks of vermiculite glisten.

— SNUG LITTLE TURBAN, WHICH HELPS
ENORMOUSLY, AS THE BALD HEAD WAS MAKING
ME VERY COLD, ESPECIALLY IF I WAS IN ANY
KIND OF BREEZE.

I wore my thinnest khakis and lightest shirt so I would
weigh less and be apportioned less of the poison red
Kool-Aid.

WON'T SCARE S— SO MUCH IF I PUT IT ON
NEXT SKYPE.

Slippery dental chair (designed for Big & Tall Men).

Bags of IV hung on racks.

Anti-nausea (pro-constipation) meds.

TRYING OUT FOR THE LEAD IN 'WIT'
TOMORROW.

Cold, cold red cocktail through my veins; two pairs of
socks and a winter hat in the middle of June.

My nurse C— donned a haz-mat smock and gloves
before shooting me up, three syringes down the clavicle.

Beads in tubing collected, merged —

Giant, slippery dental chair beneath two layers of heated white clinic blankets.

I drank liter after liter of bottled water to flush— flush— and (Constipation Wars) <u>hydrate</u> —

RESTLESSNESS (repetitive motions such as —

Multiple excursions to the restroom hauling the IV past cubicles of patients in giant dental chairs or beds; tables of unfinished jigsaw puzzles; racks of donated knit hats; the kitchenette of coffees and teas, waters and juices, salads and sandwiches — *help yourself* —

URINE DECREASE (tea-colored, concentrated)

— date stenciled —

LOVE AND MEMORIES

— check of lungs beneath and through my shirt (cool stethoscope —

I shivered; watch-checked; flipped through *New Yorkers* and *Vanity Fairs* —

I thought I had more time.

Early attempts to shit a cement pinecone resulted in a small but perilous (skull and crossbones white count) bleeding rupture and a hastily amended regimen: pails of beach sand Miralax swirled into glasses of tepid sewer swill; handfuls of tiny red coated stool softeners;

sitz bath stews in a cheap plastic tub; panicked, OCD apprehension of every morsel and every sip of liquid ingested over the next six months; daily morning Terror on the Toilet —

I thought I had —

— ineffective prunes, syrupy prune juice, sour flax oil —

ONE INFUSION AHEAD OF ME, AS WE LIKE TO
KEEP —

Prunes, much enjoyed in civilian life, morphed into the disgusting and —

FRENCH OPEN HAS ARRIVED TO DISTRACT US
FROM THE POSSIBILITY THAT WE BOTH COULD
BE —

- stomach pain
- diarrhea

Disconnect to what I ate, attributed solely to the "anti-emetics". Nausea vs. constipation —

- increased thirst

Food as disgustitude (chocolate to a chocoholic —

- appetite changes

Only frightful doses of Miralax, stool softeners, and vats of tepid sewer swill before, during and after —

- low white blood cell count
- risk of bleeding from low platelet count

Pink Cup, Blue Cup —

- nail changes
- hair loss
- nausea
- vomiting

Heat wave, flirting with 90°; her lime and white-striped tee-shirt —

- weight gain or loss
- mouth and throat sores

Stripes do camouflage Flat Chest, through I draw glances wherever I —

- heart problems

I disconcert.

- temporary or permanent cessation of menstrual —

Heat wave and huge black stain along the wall above the *Dwarf Siberian* kale seedlings. Upon closer inspection the stain shimmers and reveals itself to be a mass of tiny ants, a buggy hairpiece in motion.

- unusual tiredness or weakness

A million slide down the wall and descend on the two
seedlings. Hose gush floods plants and ants alike.
They swirl and regroup in the puddle, swarming over
leaves and stems, soggy seedlings face down in the mud.
A few more desperate gushes deepen the puddle with no
discernible impact.

- dizziness

This morning, no trace of ants; kale no worse for wear?

- separation of fingernail or toenail from the nail
  bed

Brown and black striped chipmunk disappears in a crack
in the wall.

- eye pain

Arugula by the daffodils!

- itchy, red, watery, or irritated eyes

— stenciled in: *2013*

— TO START A GARDEN —

'5th Avenue' perfume on the dresser —

- pain, burning, or tingling in the hands or feet

Large hospital Ziploc labeled: *1 yellow wedding band*

... silk stockings, pair of white gloves (?); jewelry; two heirloom rosaries (one beaded brown, the other clear); antique pocket watch (Pépère's?); initialed lace handkerchiefs; packs of Bicycle Standard playing cards; soft glasses cases; black leather gloves; scarves and belts ...

- red discoloration of urine (for 1 to 2 days after dose)

... two booklets (from my father's time — my sister's?) on grieving, *My Friend, I Care*; on dying, *Gone from My Sight*; purple velvet sack with my father's wedding band; many pairs of lovely earrings; sets of pajamas: three winter, three summer, a cute blue pair with tumbling sheep (not the kind of whimsy I would associate with —

- hives
- skin rash
- itching

... handwritten notes, page after page dealing with the bureaucracy of widowhood — whom she talked to on such and such a date, a skeptical — *Ha* —penned in beside something 'promised in the mail' —

- difficulty breathing or swallowing

... his glasses and wallet;. guest book from his wake; obituary clippings; leather Bible filled with funeral cards...

"To a swell mate who really puts volume in her voice."

~Luck, Connie

Two maroon and white yearbooks.

"Best of luck to a fellow Woolworth's laborer."

~ Rochelle

"Good luck with all your love affairs." ~ Gus

... three metal crucifixes of varying clunkiness, assumed inherited after Mémère's or Pépère's deaths?

"Be a good girl or I'll spank you." ~ Henry

— plastic half-cylinder, threaded with fat rope, for *putting on socks* —

(I've never seen these.)

Seedlings unmolested.

Trio of coyote urine capsules on the grass?

Arugula bounces up, cluster of cloverish *cotyledons* —

— miracle —

"What's the matter with your Red Sox?" ~ Gene

One ant-bombed *Dwarf Siberian* kale stripped to stem, yet alive.

— sewage, sipped at room temperature through a straw, the only way to choke down sufficient quantities.

Her Pink — my Blue plastic water cups — gagged — filled — refilled —

The other, unaffected?

— *inexorable sadness of plastic* —

Counted ounces; counted cups —

— all summer, to distract us from (sharpness on the left side of the head equals —

... bag of *Lifesaver* mints; handful of sterile 'artificial skin' wipes; anti-fungal cream; tube of *Vaseline*; cheap watch; pink nightie slit up the back ; underwear and socks ...

... daybook from 2009 with my father's appointments annotated, then my mother's as she moved into widowhood (careful recording of the car's mileage, the need for oil changes —

My aunt leaves a small pot of geraniums and lilies graveside for her sister, her brother-in-law, her parents—

My nephew reports that the location is *beautiful*, the setting sun.

Four pairs of pajamas back to New Hampshire, the summer ones with the tumbling sheep.

Slowly, the closet —

Quick spin on the highway to keep the battery from dying again. The car smells of my father though he's been gone almost four years.

Big Band CDs rattle around the side pockets.

Two more pairs of her glasses, one for driving, one wrap-around sunglasses, taken after my sister's death. Inspection stickers long expired.

Cherry Coffee Cake recipe (distinct Catholic penmanship) has remained, untouched, on the breadbox. I pass the card to my brother, for whom she intended this favorite cake at the holidays, along with the can of cherries from the closet.

> DO SOMETHING LOVELY THIS WEEKEND AND WRITE ME ABOUT IT SO I CAN LIVE VICARIOUSLY.

— homemade pie dough mix in a Tupperware container, three sticks of 'real' butter for her anticipated holiday —

She was able to make her Christmas fudge, though we couldn't find Pépère's long-handled wooden spoon and she had to use a much shorter one.

Grass filling in across the rectangle.

The fudge was perfect as ever.

Pot of bright red geraniums and day lilies.

She froze a small package, wrapped in foil, without possibly knowing we would share this last batch after her service — not six weeks —

Deterrents: *human hair* —

— grenade of moistened coyote-urine pellets, then I maneuver the Ziploc of clipped brown curls, with the aid of the 'Reacher', over the wall and flip the bag as close to the hole as I can.

Fat robin —

No 'chucks lately, though rumored to have relocated behind the rhododendron in the upper yard, the Bermuda Triangle where four neighbor properties converge in a fence post.

Some trauma, perhaps from the $34°$ night; yellowing leaves. I am less and less —

Fat robin, frozen fence statue —

Pop of heat, $90°$ predicted. (I'm leaving for a week.)

I work my morning's organic coffee grounds gently around the base of the *Black Beauty* zucchini and a *Boston Pickling* with the baby pitchfork, hoping to ameliorate whatever ails.

Chipmunks gambol over the upper moss-bog —

I suspect they'll welcome the heat.

— thunderstorms, possible 'heavy hail', 'wind damage', breaks of sun, temperatures in the 70s, climbing to 90° for a three-day —

> FOLKS HERE ACKNOWLEDGE: 'IT USUALLY DOESN'T GO UP SO HIGH.' 'LET'S WAIT AND SEE.' 'STAY AWAY FROM CHINESE BUFFETS.'

Neglected mouth (eighteen months), plaque and tartar —

> COLLECTIVE HEAD SCRATCHING, AS THOUGH THEY'VE NEVER SEEN SUCH —

- seizures
- joint pain
- pain in the lower back/side/stomach/abdomen

After the third infusion I developed ulcerations — pink lines or welts — along the sides of and beneath my tongue.

> — PAINFUL LESIONS ON MY TONGUE AND GUMS MAKING EATING, DRINKING AND EVEN TALKING CHALLENGING AND AT TIMES EXCRUCIATING TO THE POINT OF TEARS.

Single spoonful of pureed lentil soup, jagged bits of cumin seed (shards of glass) against the —

NO WAY TO TREAT OTHER THAN OFFER THIS
'MAGIC MOUTHWASH' WHICH NUMBS UP THE
AREA VERY BRIEFLY SO I CAN ATTEMPT TO
SLOWLY AND CAREFULLY CHEW SOME SOFT
FOOD WITHOUT CRYING IN AGONY.

I rushed to the sink to spit the mouthful and rinse (screaming, hearing myself scream —

Liquid (eating, speaking, swallowing, speaking —

— SO TERRIFIC THROUGH THIS ORDEAL—

I obtained a pink Pepto-Bismol prescription called *Magic Mouthwash* to numb the region and allow food to pass. The mouthwash numbed my lips, tongue and teeth like Novocain.

I tried to place a small piece of pasta in a sore-free region of my mouth and chew very, very carefully.

The mouthwash wore off fast and I would aggravate the numbed sores because I couldn't feel what I was —

Hold your loved one's –

Trials and errors and liquid —

Repetitive smoothies made with peaches and almond milk, protein shakes, vanilla extract and crushed —

"THINGS WILL GET BETTER."

A good soul on one of the sites recommended q-tips for this malady, so I dipped the pink goo, painted only the lesions themselves, and tried to eat quickly before the numbness wore off.

Straws helped, if positioned just right through the buccal landmine.

Pale, paleness; fear of transfusion —

- cough or hoarseness
- flushing of face

— probiotics in a white bottle —

> ATE YOUR PASTA AGAIN AND MADE STRAWBERRY SMOOTHIES WITH YOUR STRAWBERRIES —

— mortality, a significantly high percentage —

> AGAIN AT THE POINT OF STOPPING —

... sister (breast); mother (breast, colon); father (lymphoma) ...

— eyelids slightly open —

... uncle (brain); great-aunts (breast, breast); uncle (pancreas); uncle (prostate) ...

— pupils enlarged, eyes fixed on a certain —

... aunt (leukemia); aunt (not specified); grandfather (not specified – stomach?) ; cousin (kidney); cousin (melanoma) ...

— just to taste the ice cream (scream and rush to the —

> "Fever that is 100.4° or higher for more than one hour, or a one time temperature of 101° or higher."

Manic thermometer beeps indicated DANGER —

— day when there are no new sensations —

- painful/difficult urination

We drove to the 24-hour pharmacy, midnight odyssey through deserted streets and flashing —

> "Call your doctor right away, even if this happens in the middle of the night."

Blackbirds (sparrows, finches, maybe a crow or two?) gone bonkers — cawking and frenzied fluttering across the lawn between the *Boston Picklings*, combing the neighbor's lawn, pecking some delicacy that spontaneously materialized within the last ten minutes.

> — OVER THE WEEKEND, THEN FEVER MONDAY NIGHT, FOLLOWED BY —

Grass — lilac — fence — sputtering — zipping along wall — fence —grass — zooming through the shade of the maple —

"ORAL MUCOSITIS"

— beaks ravage — peck-pecking — bacchanalia of yellow beaks —

— TRULY GRATEFUL —

Mr. W reconnoiters at the *Boston Picklings* by the daisies. When I rap on the window he lopes away, nonchalant, daring me to stand sentry all night in the sunporch.

— beginnings of the end (?) of my Noble —

Dare I?

Blackbirds regroup, howling monkeys —

Fluffy, fuchsia, seven-foot bouquet where the fences meet, surpassing the neighbor's rose-red —

Everywhere bold, bold yellow — *Eat me* — blossoms (a wonder how anything —

— birds having birthed (hatched)?

Birdy block party celebrating the arrival of —

Speak gently.

90° and North Carolina tomorrow, my first vacation in two years.

Anticipating the party in my absence: Chip 'n Dale, Mr. W and extended family, drunken birds, master race squirrels, what could possibly —

They, too, are spectacular.

I take a field trip to round out the herb bed: dill, *Thai* basil, *Lemon Thai* basil seedlings from an organic farm in South County.

— *Jalapeño* starts — a gift — with a few mint —

Prodigious rains in the night produce plump yellow blossoms on the *Black Beauty* zukes along the fence. Yellow bells wide open for a few hours.

First furred, doll-sized pickle behind a yellow cuke blossom!

Rains or warmth or combination?

Everything snapping to attention — even the mud-spattered kale and the half-drowned *Thai* basil —

Birdy block party dissipates or relocates to another, more happenin' lawn. Cacophony reduced to single bleating from high in the —

Perfect still night.

Cicadas — cicadas — cicadas —

— cacti dormant —

(The hydroponic, hairy-rooted transplants are a bust.)

High, high —

Darkness descends, day unmarked beyond the churned
batch of vanilla ice cream; the tended garden; the
postponed tennis match on television; the stroll around
the block (*gorgeous* rhododendrons on parade); the
carefully wedged air conditioner into the upstairs
window (imagined pitch to the driveway below, the
crushed Honda hood —

6:12 AM, impossibility in the soupy sweatbox, night of
storms —

Bookcase of photo albums on the floor in the hallway,
many binders.

> "DUE TO SOME VERY RECENT UNFORESEEN
> CIRCUMSTANCES —"

Had I known Mémère was a *flapper*?

> "I'VE DECIDED TO SUSPEND MY SEARCH THIS
> YEAR—"

— inspection, and The Garden stands, though some
leaves gnawed clean. One cuke and one zuke.

New leaves emerge. More doll-sized pickles behind
spindly shoots.

Corner arugula soldiers on thickly, incognito —

Some shriveled, indifferent blossoms.

Basil steady.

Thai basil flowers again — purple.

Jalapeño ears flap, annoyed, in the breeze.

Slo-Bolt cilantro too crowded. Weed, and thin, when I get
some —

- black/tarry stools
- bloody mucus in stools

Fur balls writhing everywhere, undeterred by the freshly
scalped (lowest possible wheel setting) lawn.

Two babies loiter, brazen, outside the entry.

- fast/irregular heartbeat

When I crack the door they scamper down the walkway
beneath the gutters, and wriggle through a hole in the
tool shed against the house.

- shortness of breath

Improvised concoction: old mehti (fenugreek) seeds from my spice stash; dash of cayenne; heavy sprinkle of garlic powder; teaspoons each of natural dish detergent and vegetable oil. Add water; strain into mister; spritz brown sludge onto cuke, zuke, basil leaves —

- swelling of ankles/feet

I cannot pass the sunporch without spying two or three furballs shuffling along the upper yard, mowing through millimeters of mangled clover.

How anything — any leaf, stem, green thing (ants, beetles, spiders, worms, birds —

Pollinate (eat) me —

— maple-compromised — now the leaves —

Do I *dare Disturb* —

Shiny cemetery ivy brushes the front yard —

Rather than retreat over the wall to their burrow, they opt to flatten their bodies, stick their bums in the air like skunks, and merge into the shadowy, moss-covered tool shed corners.

Clang of rusted hoe on cement floor produces no effect.

In an effort to deter shed denizens, I drop a single pricey urine pellet and water with the watering can to disgorge its gelatinous contents.

A few short weeks and the seeded expansion has produced its golf course for the future departed (morning obituary of Mr. P— , father of a childhood friend, same hospice as my —

— photos from Rehoboth, breeze blowing colored kites behind our (how we could — not *two years* —

Geraniums against the stone, still bright, cheerful with all the rains —

Chipmunk and the Robin —

— with the magic vacuum-mower, to decapitate a mouse by the spent daffodils, or more specifically — 'bifurcate' — 'disembowel'— what was once a creature with a long, mouse-ish tail.

BREATHING PATTERN CHANGE

Flies descend on the entrails hidden in the grass.

Two hours: scraped out threads of grass from between the *Genovese* basil; loosened rain-sodden dirt around the rosemary and thyme; separated and thinned *Giant of Italy* parsley and *Slo-Bolt* cilantro shoots, relocating the most robust to patches with space to breathe; marveled at the *Boston Pickling* doll-pickles hiding under leaves; hunted for new yellow blossoms; pruned lilac runners and a few branches of reachable maple to allow a bit more light along the fence.

(I am sorry.)

> — SUGGESTED MY VEINS WERE SMALL AND I MUST HAVE A PORT. THE PROCEDURE FAILED.

Zukes and cukes along the wall look particularly dreary though green leaves emerge.

> THE VEINS KEPT COLLAPSING AND THE SURGEON SUGGESTED THAT THIS HAD NEVER HAPPENED TO HIM BEFORE.

All trying to maintain; lean into light.

> I WAS SENT HOME WITH MULTIPLE PRICKS AND HOLES THROUGHOUT MY CHEST AND NECK, DIFFICULTY SWALLOWING AND A SEVERE BACKACHE, KEEPING ME FROM TAKING A DEEP BREATH.

Russet maple drips rain.

> HAD TO SPEND THE NIGHT IN A RECLINER BECAUSE I COULD NOT LIE FLAT.

— coiling ivy climbs the stoop and pushes through the top of the azaleas —

> STILL CANNOT TAKE A DEEP BREATH AND AM TAKING EXTRA STRENGTH TYLENOL TO MANAGE—

Caveat emptor (fifty years in my parents' capable —

... tables and chairs; sofas; recliners; hutch; desks; beds; mirrors; bureaus; dishes; glasses; pots; pans; appliances; televisions; air conditioners; fans; luggage; Christmas decorations; clothes.

Hallway closet of Amazing Technicolor Coats.

(She never did get to use the fluffy lemon bathmat ordered online, her last purchase —

I ran into Dr. Port Failure repeatedly, dragging my IV to the ladies room; in hallways; waiting for the elevator; and made a point to avoid eye contact. For some reason he seemed to want to —

— **no blinking** —

— holes pocked through my bruised chest on either side of the sternum. I could neither inhale deeply nor move without pain slicing through my —

— **jaw relaxed** —

I bumbled downstairs, arranged myself in a recliner in the den, and attempted to fall asleep for many, many —

— **mouth slightly open** —

Rearranged ... arranged ... marking every inhalation —
exhalation —

X-rays confirmed the partially collapsed ("rare" *blah blah,*
"less than 5%" *blah blah)* lung —

Your veins are *very tiny.*

Tiny veins.

Tiny, very tiny.

Never happened to me before!

After a semi-emergency trip to Boston, vascular
specialists implanted the port beneath my left clavicle the
following morning without incident.

— *so sorry* —

The elevator descent was a bewildering coal mine
journey of many, many minutes, or was it the sedation;
the operating room was, again, an icicle.

> IMMEDIATELY MADE A DERMATOLOGY
> APPOINTMENT, SO THAT'S WHERE WE'RE
> HEADED.

I said to the nurses *it feels like snow.*

> (INSERT EXPLETIVE OF YOUR CHOICE HERE).

Father's Day at Resurrection.

Mourners in pairs, families, gather graveside. Arms across one another's backs.

Stone and grass —

Geraniums looking well in their clay pot with all the rain.

Sometimes they flop to the ground, picnic-like, *sans* food.

> ROUTINE FOLLOW-UP AT THE SURGEON'S
> OFFICE. REMOVED REMAINING STERI-STRIPS,
> LIFTED ALL RESTRICTIONS, SUGGESTED A CANE
> FOR THE REST OF HER —

Four months and the grave has reseeded, the clipped grass blending seamlessly with *Our Town* neighbors in every direction.

> ... DOZING ALL DAY...

Pansies, violets, petunias proliferate. Tall white racks hold the most recent arrangements, shoulder to shoulder.

Lilies begin to sag.

The canopy of red maple leaves filters most mid-afternoon sun from the fence seedlings; a few green leaves and the odd yellow blossom but mostly stunted, moribund, waterlogged by recent deluges.

Baby doll pickles as big as my thumb appear — drop off—

(I WOULD BE VERY SURPRISED IF THE SCAN
DIDN'T —

— large random basil bites —

A few feathery, improbable carrot tops.

I thin the arugula with kitchen shears and toss a handful
into my tarragon chickpea frittata.

— quite scarce since the tool shed escapade.
Coincidence? Or have they set out to establish their own
burrows, being, as I read, 'solitary creatures'.

Boo-wee — *boo-wee* — *boo-wee* from the fence rail: elegy;
invitation; love song; paean to the cool, overcast day and
the neighbor's newly mown lawn, the crop of unwitting
worms tunneling to the surface.

— ball in the net from the bottom of the driveway in his
three-piece suit. (When I explained we could no longer
lift him in and out of the wheelchair, that he would have
to move into the hospice facility, he nodded and seemed
to understand.)

— more rain —

— yard work in his checked shorts, <u>black</u> socks —

In the freezer were her last batch of fudge, her *Sally Lunn*
rolls, and a carrot cake for Christmas.

Intended, never completed holiday recipes in a rubber-banded bundle on top of the bread box: *Cherry Coffee Cake, Sweet Potato Casserole, Black & Gold Marble Cake, Xmas Butter Cookies, French Apple Pie* —

— her death — my —

Train-track stitches, lines of looped, black thread-gut —

BEST STRATEGY IS NOT TO —

— last tub of her refrigerated pie dough mix (flour, Crisco, salt) —

Black train-tracks held my chest(s) together.

— share, distribute, discard (necessity of making even a simple —

Cherry Coffee Cake recipe (distinct Catholic penmanship) to my —

... fans; air conditioners; books; needlepoint; beds; tools; paints; filing cabinets; shoes; coats; Christmas ornaments; mirrors; blender; Dutch oven; toaster-oven; food processor; televisions; radios; pocketbooks; sheets; towels; blankets; quilts; pillows; air mattresses; lawn mower; buckets; bookcases; books; lamps; laptop; toys; phones; canned goods; flour tin; sugar tin; china; wine glasses; popcorn popper; candlesticks; photo albums; hammers; vacuum; broom; mop; prescriptions; glasses ...

— tingling along the top of my —

Five whole around Resurrection —

Dud dill transplant — instant wilt.

Unable to read.

Can one return dud (dead) plants?

— the transition with support, understanding and ease.

Quank—quank rehearsal —

HYPONATREMIA (VERY LOW SODIUM WHICH CAN CAUSE A WHOLE HOST OF ALARMING —

For some reason the operating room was an icicle. I said —

WE'RE HOPING THIS IS ALL—

Other discharge goodies: hospital-stamped pink Red Sox cap; two generic prosthetic bras with spongy, pillowish inserts —

— PATHOLOGY REPORT AND THE SKIN METASTASIS IS NOT FROM THE COLON BUT SECONDARY TO —

Despite making my intentions clear both before and after the surgery that I would not reconstruct, I was treated as though this baffling whim would surely —

... bedding towels; mattresses; mirrors; bureaus; bookcases; glasses; plates; bowls; pots; pans; cookie sheets; pie plates; cake tins; knives; Tupperware; spices; canned goods; wet-vac ...

Drains dripped bloody chunks into dangling rubber bulbs, one for each excised breast.

... bed frames; box springs; photo albums; frames; photos; filing cabinets; cables; decorative glass; pitchers; wine glasses ...

Two white Velcro camisoles were dispatched upon discharge.

... candlesticks; china; goblets; coffee maker; toaster oven; files; records; papers; snow shovels ...

Drain-bulbs sat in drain pockets.

Plastic tubes connected wounds to bulbs.

... bags of vintage mittens; hats; scarves ...

I slept on my back, wary of squishing, crushing or tangling the blood-chunk tubing. I emptied the bulbs into a white lab beaker several times a day, recorded the volume, and flushed the blood- chunks down the toilet.

— again, shortness of breath at the top of the —

The complimentary spongy prosthesis rode up on my flat chest and was not especially comfortable.

Final impulse spree at the garden store —

The as yet unfilled year-old prescription for a 'fitted' prosthesis is somewhere among the piles of medical bills, pamphlets, records —

I prefer —

: three heirloom tomato plants (two *Yellow Pear* and one *Black Krim*); two clay pots; one bag of organic potting soil from Maine; one red and one green pepper plant.

All, as of two hours ago, planted in ground, basket or pot, eased into the world on this rare 80° sunny spring day on the verge of summer solstice.

Dwarf Siberian kale good cheer, defying the wall infestation.

Anemic cukes and zukes strain to put forth one or two blossoms, flapping in and out of maple's shadows.
Dud dill either (a) eaten overnight, victim of beetles, chipmunks, birds, Tan Bunny ... ?

Serrano Tampiqueno begin to take hold, thanks to the tease of heat.

— ENTER —

Arugula impervious to the ant lode streaming out of the
wall, swamping the stems.

— search terms — "BARTLETT —

> *Joseph Bartlett: 1715-1791*
> *Jacob B. Sweet, 1789-1871*
> *Lydia Cook Sweet, 1790-1858*

Cemetery branches brush the second floor bedroom
windows.

> *"Many persons have been eulogized for*
> *their great and good deeds, yet few have*
> *left behind them such an enviable*
> *reputation —"*

Homeruns on the fly or one bounce from the street into
this jungle —

> *"HISTORICAL CEMETERY,*
> *BARTLETT LOT. 75' x 50' in poor*
> *condition; no enclosure."*

I slide open the dusty screen, seize a leaf, squeeze the
pruning shears and release one branch, then another,
some twenty feet to the mossy lawn below.

"Extensively overgrown with weeds,
briars, and trees."

Whiffleball shots from our tiny yard, over the wall, into
the —

"Many stones down, broken or missing."

Tan Bunny darts out of the forsythia to nibble clover —

"Neighbor dumping washing machine
waste into cemetery."

— darts back when I crack the screen door —

"Willis Jillson, 1819-1832, unfortunately
killed by being thrown from a horse May
19, 1832, in the 14th year of his life."

— rubber-coasted blasts lofted from the J—'s back yard
over Bartlett Street, into the forbidding forest. No one
wanted to retrieve the ball in the poison ivy overgrowth,
but someone always —

Children: Abel Bartlett, Chloe Bartlett,
Jacob Bartlett, Abner Bartlett, Levinia
Bartlett, Phebe Bartlett, Joseph Bartlett ...

I also prune the forsythia underbrush along the of
driveway, squeezing the shears with all my might to snap
some of the thicker branches; scattering many, many
pounds of leaf debris to the cement; filling two giant

paper lawn refuse bags (hoping the bunnies henceforth
might avoid the clipped, aerated forsythia and their
favored clover buffet, three feet from the demolished dill,
the tattered kale along the side of the —

"Estimated 30 burials from 1715-1871."

'chuck! Welcome back!

Eliza Cook Sweet, 1816-1822

One of the babies grazes clover on the neighbor's lawn
then scoots back to the rhododendron Bermuda Triangle
upon screen door squeak.

What killed poor 6-year-old Eliza.

— burst, then trickle of hand-addressed, pastel
envelopes—

> *" — probity of conduct as is credited to the*
> *good, earnest, pious old Quaker —"*

He can't but apprehend along his route, house by house
(hospitals, Medicare, hospice, insurance, month after —

Post-twilight thunderstorm.

—TLC catalogs —

I creep among the borders in my pjs, scattering scoopfuls
of donated 'Critter Ridder' thither and yon.

— left throat ... (enlarged node?)

— one side — both sides —

The dying person might experience varied and mixed —

Nothing.

Nothing.

Black Krim heirloom tomato —

Ticklish sensation —

Teeth cleaning; credit union; simple will; boxes of books and papers in the basement; Curly Temple bouffant haircut —

Nothing?

Clearing more than usual?

Mowing — like vacuuming!

PLEASE. NO PHONE CALLS.

— in odd flippy curls again.

I LOVE YOU ALL.

Disheartening. I do not want odd flippy —

Leave valuables at home. Wear comfortable clothing. Arrange for a driver.

IF IT IS MY TIME TO GO, I AM AT PEACE.

Leave the steri-strips in place. They will fall off on their own. This can take up to 10-14 days.

— ANY MINUTE AFTER HER 10-DAY HOSPITAL VENTURE —

The breast tissue has been sewn together and will heal.

— DOWN THE RABBIT HOLE —

Do not worry if the steri-strips fall off. Your wound will not open.

"YOU ARE IN OUR PRAYERS."

Post-mow, prompt shower with clothes and garden gloves in the washing machine to outwit any poison—

Your stay at the hospital has been listed as 'one night' admission, although that is very much up to the discretion of the –

— "spreading oils with water"? I anticipate outbreaks any minute on arms, face, places where dew from the forsythia branches splashed —

— has mailed me *Interpreter of Maladies*. (The title alone.)

149

— days, weeks, months, the least in a lifetime of reading.

Heavy-lidded; cotton-brained.

Missing sinking my brain into a good, crisp read.

I request the new *Selected Letters of Willa Cather* from the library, sanguine —

... AT PEACE WITH THIS IF...

3:17 AM podcast discussion of 'end of life' care. A caller suggests that we have unrealistic expectations about what doctors, drugs and technology can do in the face of terminal illness.

Another caller suggests that in his experience with hospice, both patients and families end up insisting that 'everything possible' be done, rejecting the credo of comfort and acceptance, not prolonging the dying —

Robin — fence post —

First day of summer —

The host, a septuagenarian, tackles these issues far more often than any other program.

This month's e-bulletin: *Summer Smarts and Cancer.*

Choosing a Wig.

Left neck beneath the jawbone.

What Every Woman Should Know.

Noticeable difference from right side (though more 'sensation' — nothing palpable —

Considering a Clinical Trial. Boost Your Immune System with Leafy —

Turning point? Beginning of 'active' —

> TRYING TO ADJUST TO THE NEW, MUTILATED
> ME.

Clear, clearing throat (high pollen count —

> (THE BEST STRATEGY IS NOT TO LOOK IN THE—

— many boxes (current 'proxy'?) to cull, weed, organize—

> — LIKE I HAVE THE FLU —

Summer tomorrow. Warm weather rushes in, with more intense sun.

Boo-wee — boo-wee — quank-quank —

> ... ENORMOUS, ENORMOUS ...

Dwarf Siberian kale doubles overnight, rebounding after last month's ant barrage.

Genovese basil stretches towards the —

(High pollen?)

"— HUGS ACROSS —"

Jalapeño flowers in cute white blossoms which droop upside-down. Is this —

— rosemary (herb plot-snipped) golden raisin oatmeal toast —

Cemetery trees scrape and brush the upstairs windows.

'White ash'? 'Elm'? (internet as poor reference —

— MOUNTAIN IN THE DRIVEWAY HANGS ON —

I stake the *Yellow Pear* and the *Black Krim* in their terracotta pots with assorted steel poles found in a cobweb corner of the garage. (My father's horde or simply too long for any trash receptacle?)

— EVERY DAY, MANY TIMES A DAY...

"Old panty hose" (top bureau) make fine ties, as they are "kind to vines".

"... PRAYERS, LOVE, AND GOOD KARMA ..."

In the aisles, strangers' eyes flutter toward and away from my — concavities —

Not bird-watching, but *vegetable* watching with the cheap field glasses on the table in the sunporch.

— hands in her blue garden gloves —

LOST A MONTH SOMEWHERE —

Trying to catch a growth spurt through the screen —

Brown gloves on top of the breadbox. She put these on to take anything out of the freezer and would not let me do that for her. She wore them in the market, too, the cold and frozen food aisles.

FUN FOR THE DAY WAS LEARNING TO SET
MOUSETRAPS.

I held her hand bedside, something I hadn't done since I was probably 4-years-old.

A SMALL ONE SLITHERED ACROSS THE LIVING
ROOM LAST NIGHT WHILE WE WERE WATCHING
PROJECT RUNWAY.

I rubbed them with nice-smelling lotion.

... QUE SERA, SERA ...

She was awake ... asleep ... I sat by the bed and held the hand closest to —

NEUROPATHY, BUT WE'RE HOPING THAT WILL —

Bony; warm; dry.

— MICE IN THE CELLAR, FOUR AS OF THIS
MORNING, IN CHEAP BUT EFFECTIVE LITTLE
WOODEN —

Knuckles swollen (her wedding band removed before the
last surgery, sent home in a clear plastic —

— CANNOT THINK VERY —

— his hand, too, minutes before he departed, though he
was not conscious, and could not squeeze my hand when
I —

ALL QUIET ON THE EASTERN FRONT.

(She phoned and called me 'Farmer MacGregor'.)

HAVEN'T REGAINED MY APPETITE FOR —

Every two hours the lights flicked on and a nurse,
apologetic, came in to take blood pressure, pulse ox,
temperature —

— center of gravity — an immediate —

— left throat with the backs of my left —

> "... SITTING IN PEET'S ON VAN NESS - IT'S 6:50
> AM AND THE MORNING SUN IS ANGLING IN THE
> WINDOW. EVERYONE IN THE PLACE IS READING
> SOMETHING OR OTHER."

Feeling only (wishful ignorance —

"PLEASE TELL ME ABOUT YOUR CURRENT STATE OF HEALTH."

Silence across the yard.

"I DO VERY MUCH WANT YOU TO SURVIVE."

Awake and up at 5:35 AM, summer —

Hand in hand —

"YES, MY BASIL GREW TO BE AN ENORMOUS HEIGHT THERE IN BUCK'S COUNTY."

Holding my toddler niece's —

"THE SOIL WAS VIRGIN BLACK AND EVERYTHING GREW HIGH. LIKE THE LINE IN THE WALLACE STEVENS POEM ABOUT FLORIDA'S 'VENEREAL' SOIL."

Speak gently.

His hand, too, was cool and dry.

Yes, San Francisco in the fall, should the stars — the cosmic —

Heavy.

ENORMOUS STRESS ON HER, AS YOU CAN IMAGINE, THOSE 'NADIR' DAYS BEFORE MY COUNTS BEGIN TO —

Nine years since my last visit. I flew home mid-August to my sister's hospice, her second floor bedroom. We chatted about my vacation. I said I ate and drank to excess.

She said *that's what vacations are for*.

> — PALLIATIVE AND LET ME SLIP AWAY TO THE *GRAND* —

She was hard to make out, her voice was so —

Maybe —

— to the bathroom but was clumsy, misunderstanding her directions how to plant myself and brace my arms beneath her arms to help her rise —

> — A CRAPSHOOT—

Downstairs I had a meltdown in the dining room.

Spectacular blue sky, low humidity.

Longest —

I never again saw her conscious.

Finches? Wrens? Chickadees? Thrushes?

Fog over the Bridge, and falling asleep to foghorns.

Walking the wide busy sidewalks.

I know my sparrows, robins, blue jays, cardinals, pigeons
(unhelpful, decrepit *Birds of North America Guidebook* in
the magazine rack —

Even the hilly-hills, though I could scarcely tackle them
these days.

— up insects across the newly mown lawn. Baby
sparrows on the fencepost.

Eliza Cook Sweet, 1816-1822

Riotous pre-dawn *dwee-buh-dee - dwee- dwee* —

The beige bird with the long tail pecking through the
neighbor's grass is def a *mourning dove.*

("I prefer not to.")

Dwee- dwee — *quank-quank* —

Proliferation of robins across the stone border.

*"Note the slim body and long tapered tail. Flight is swift and
direct, without coasting; the whistling of the wings is
diagnostic."*

Expressionless, not unlike cats I have known.

"Call, ooah-ooo-oo-oo, 4-6, minute ..."

Pinch the purple buds on the *Thai* basil —

"Their soft, drawn-out calls sound like laments."

To honor the summer solstice, a batch of strawberry ice cream with a quart of fresh picked strawberries from Cooks Valley ('since 1705') Farm.

— to ignore — ignore —

Nothing.

> — WHILE YOU'RE SIGNING THE LOVELY '/
> *CONSENT TO BE POISONED'* FORM —

Some of these very same Cook ancestors are buried next door over the wall.

— sensation of difference in the cords of my left —

— 'chucks winding in and out of their mould —

Left neck — right —

Left —

Humidity rising, 'Cool Breeze' fan working overtime.

Left —

The anemic cukes and zukes have glorious yellow 'bell' blossoms, but few new leaves and no vine growth.

— crossing over —

Rootbound transplants?

Two direct-seeded *Boston Pickling* cukes have popped along the wall, green *cotyledons* flaring.

Refusal to cross —

> "... with this type of medication have developed
> other cancers (e.g., secondary leukemia) ..."

Left — right —

"I prefer not —

Jam session high in the maple —

The medical assistant who called my name (out-of-town, out-of- state clinic) turned out to be L— , a neighbor who grew up four houses from us, sister of my late sister's best childhood friend.

She lost two brothers and her mother to cancer.

Raspberries bleed through the cardboard box onto my white pants as I twist and weave between the rows, oblivious, for plumper, more perfect —

We speculated briefly about possible —

— my lightest pants, my thinnest —

Weight; pulse ox; blood pressure —

— like some terrible wound — gunshot to my inner
thigh—

— as low as 110 (which I hadn't weighed since I was in
elementary school —

— buttony bump (peach pit) under the skin of my left
clavicle. She located the port bump with her fingers,
though it was clearly —

Syringes of 'Red Devil' pink antifreeze were plunged
manually —port to jugular — by my nurse in her haz-
mat—

"— sores on the lips, mouth and throat may —"

Bags of 'anti-emetics' on a steel pole —

"— limit hot foods and drinks, brush your teeth
carefully, avoid using mouthwash that contains
alcohol —"

— beneath two heated blankets in the dental recliner,
despite repeated pillow arranging behind my back,
against my —

When the instrumental *Memories of You* comes on the
radio, I cannot help —

— colorless drip — drip — drip —

— drip —

— drip —

— drip — drip —

— drip —

— drip —

— waiver (*yes, I understood the substantial* —

— drip —

> "... heart problems, including possibly fatal heart failure —"

Pick your poison, I said to my —

> "— during therapy or months to years after receiving —"

— difficulty getting out of bed; flu-ish feeling —

Pale white tongue as white count barometer.

What's for dinnah ...

Pale white tongue in the mirror.

—"avoid Chinese buffets" —

I crept around the house and tried to nap again an hour after I woke.

DISORIENTATION (time, place identity)

I did have perfect bald skin, the chemo 'facial'.

— months of painless blood draws from the crease in my tiny-veined left arm, while she came home from her clinic with purple welts up and down her —

Arms; legs; face. Even the stubborn callus on the bottom of my right foot.

Crotch but for a few down low. Lashes and —

— clown box straws to choke it down, or maybe to feign festiveness.

Six. Seven. Eight.

Dinner as disgusting.

One year later, sparse arms and legs.

Slow growing strays in the armpits.

Partial pube rebound.

Brows.

Head hair in the weirdest, springiest —

Half-lashes super, super slow.

— snack, snacks through the day to prevent —

Nausea of prunes and apricots; Miralax and dulcolate —
morning terror such as never —

"— infections are a major cause of morbidity and
mortality in patients who are *neutropenic* —"

— right armpit with an <u>electric</u> razor because I lack
sensation (nick or abrasion as gateway to *lymphedema*),
but I glide a cheap pink plastic razor over the numb flab
once a month or —

— acute apprehension of any and all morsels — even
liquids —

(My sister went light 'ash' with hers, too, though she
invested in a real wig.)

"— spleen may become enlarged and can
rupture —"

"I prefer not —

"— ruptured spleen can cause death —"

... *oxycodone; metronizadole; lorezapam; ondansetron;
dexamethasone; prochlorperazine; nystatin; ciprofloxacin;
Florastor; xarelto; atorvastatin; bystolic; lisinopril; atropine*
jammed in the hutch drawer —

"The spleen is located in the upper left section of your stomach area."

— mine — hers — ours —

I dropped the white, blue, pink, peach pills in her pill box: M – T – W – Th – F – Sa – Su when she could no longer manipulate —

"Call your doctor right away if you have pain in the left upper stomach area or left shoulder tip —"

The 3:30 AM alarm was for the *dexamethasone,* washed down with a few bites of Cheerios to prevent infusion anaphylaxis.

Myriad 'chat' strategies: (1) pack hands and feet in tubs of ice during infusion (2) take mega doses of B6 (3) ingest glucosamine —

"— acute respiratory distress syndrome (ARDS)"

I was able to make a dent in the first fat *The New Yorker* article until the Benadryl began —

"— emergency care right away if you have shortness of breath, trouble breathing, or a fast rate of —"

He did say to me (and this I respected) that *if we knew what worked, everyone would be* —

— up and down the corridor to pee — pee — pee — pee
again — pee —

If this is the beginning —

— pee some more —

— jawbone, neckline (nothing concrete, though palpating
with extreme —

   "— shortness of breath, wheezing, dizziness,
   swelling around the mouth or eyes, fast pulse,
   sweating, and hives —"

Are we into the summer properly — 90° and above?

Garden embraces the 'tropics'.

— is the beginning —

Baby 'chuck on the wall outside the bathroom, first
sighting in weeks.

Big gray cat ... ?

I whistle a short, lugubrious dirge, to which he listens
politely, turns and disappears into the jungle.

After one of the fleshy arm horse shots, my knees were so
weakened I was forced to grip the vanity in order to rise
from or descend to the toilet like a 90-year-old.

— sitz baths to soothe and heal the fissure (infection, sepsis, rapid —

— biweekly horse shots in the back of the arm to boost my—

— IV up and down the corridor.

The inaugural pee was bright pink in the bowl, diluted 'Red Devil'.

If so —

— with the heavy bathroom door and IV pole, wheels up over the threshold, tangled tubes beside the toilet —

If —

Sea of seniors in the lounge, the lab for blood draws, the elevator, most of the dental chairs —

— down the corridor to the kitchen, juggling two — sometimes three spring water bottles —

If this is the beginning (sensation, swollen node) then I can only —

(Bette Davis, *Dark Victory*, planting her —

NOT EVERYONE LIVES TO BE 99.

— *daffodils* —

— tepid sewage, straws from a box with a clown on the—

Spirit of 'negative (?) adventure' (not the tragedy —

Ashes to the moors —

If this is the (not abandoning —

— moors-of-Haworth scenario — ashes —

Boxes of letters, useless papers, projects, drafts,
transcripts (a good minute to retrieve this word,
beginnings of brain —

Reader, I —

— obsolete floppy disks into the brown trash or blue
recycle —

— affectionate letters from so many old —

Spirit of —

— multi-paged, double-sided, handwritten and typed,
stationery and notebook leafs and onion skin pages,
folded up into envelope upon envelope —

Ashes, ashes —

Not until after the 4th of July visit so as not to cast any shadow (unless symptoms alarm) over this possibly last quality —

Never assume the person <u>cannot hear.</u>

JULY

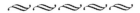

Swollen —

A robin gang has infiltrated the maple, plucking and
dropping long pale chive tubes across the lawn —

Sun-searing days near 90°.

Cuke-zukes refuse to grow, teasing out yellow females
only to languish; rot; drop.

Should I regather, rearrange —

— male to female flowers "with a small paintbrush" may
be attempted, though the vines at this point are so very—

Swollen node beneath left jawline can only (and I could
not have borne looking into her —

July (if... my final —

Maybe —

Yellow tomato blossoms begin to emerge in their respective pots.

Dwarf Siberian kale prospers.

Peppers on track.

A few scattered carrot tops.

Tan Bunny settles beneath the lilac.

'chucks AWOL.

Tepid dill rebound remains to be —

Overcast, spitting precipitation. Shut the noisy air conditioners, let the cool July air —

Dwee-buh-dee ('nest'-raising?) —

Lush lawn after all the rain, warmth, humidity. Garden starting to move and stretch, though bouncing bright kale is demolished over a two-day sneak attack, sawed down by some —

Tomato vines take off since the improvised seaweed supplement (stale nori pulverized in the coffee grinder).

Cukes and zukes tease fruit before —

FLUID AND FOOD DECREASE (wanting little or no food or fluid)

Pieces of (her) nylon stockings bind the tomato branches to a teepee of metal poles.

In the upper yard, Mr W samples daisy heads over the edge of the wall.

> — CATCHING MICE IN THE CELLAR, FOUR AS OF THIS WRITING, IN CHEAP BUT EFFECTIVE LITTLE—

Fears: —   —   —

> HOW ARE YOU FEELING IN THE LAND OF THE —

Tower of boxes: old journals; an essay for a class on my first befuddled, fog-bound summer in SF, decades ago —

> WHO KNOWS WHERE THE YEAR WENT AND WHERE IT MAY —

Studio apartment described as *"tubercular British castle that hasn't seen the sun since the 12th century"*.

Stray orange cat prowls the forsythia and scoots up the maple.

> *"I shiver and sweat alternately, trying to suppress alarming symptoms of malaria or pneumonia."*

Descends, chagrined, when I crack the screen door —

> *"I fall asleep, sock-clad, under dense winter blankets to the symphony of foghorns blasting the same tunes through my exhaustion, playing on into my dreams."*

He is astonished how close we can creep to Tan Bunny, lilac tenant.

> <u>ICD9</u>: *197.0 Secondary Malig Neo Lung*

Is she deaf? Blind?

Nonstop nibbling at whatever is on the menu at the circle patch (formerly known as our childhood 15' aluminum-sided swimming pool) buffet.

> *"I am never warm."*

Penchant for — *natch* — clover —

> *"— the deep heavy bass, the alto, the tenor, calling to each other, then in harmony.*

Weather breaks, barely; several cloudbursts.

Raggedy, holey basil resurrects and births out monster leaves overnight, one of which I pinch and toss on today's sandwich.

"4:00 AM stillness — heavy mist rolling across everything ..."

Good handful of arugula along the wall, minus the grasshopper.

Boston Pickling vine along the walk explodes in foliage.

One walnut-sized *Black Krim*; dozens of *Yellow* (green) *Pear* —

APPETITE IMPROVED.

— lone *Jalapeño* — inch and a half —

(OTHER HIDEOUS EFFECTS SO YOU DON'T GET TOO SMUG.)

Orange perennials emerge in the fecund corner; daisy heads over the wall, though 'tasty' petals soon devoured—

Brown, pigeony mourning doves, blackbirds, robins, and wrens scour the yard; alight on the fence above the cuke-zukes; poop one purple clot after —

Early morning tropics.

Baby (Young Adult) W returns after several weeks' absence, sliding along the wall and into the cemetery upon any meek half-step in his (her?) direction.

Mosquito on my shoulder too slow to suck my —

... poison; old people; wheelchairs ...

WHITE COUNT ZOOMED FROM THE LOW LAST
WEEK OF 1.5 TO 31 (OFF THE CHARTS).

... flowers; phones; clipboards and cheerful —

THE CLOCK WITH JUDY GARLAND (I REALLY
LOVED)

... hermetically sealed glass and dated cancery magazines;
unfinished jigsaw —

THE GROUP WHICH I THOUGHT WAS PRETTY
BAD, BUT DIVERSIONARY ENOUGH FOR OUR
NIGHTLY EXHAUSTED -

... blue patterned chairs. Two paper ID bracelets around
the left wrist (one for blood draw, one for onc) —

I waited and sweated, waited and sweated (AC issues?)
until I was forced to strip off my olive knit winter hat —
bald relief (patients and loved ones on the blue patterned
chairs; receptionists and clinicians; the maintenance man;
oldsters in wheelchairs trying not to glance ...

Big scars, little scars —

... failing ...

— electronically, at his fingertips, but didn't recall or
process or refresh that no, you were not *an only child* (you
are one of six), nor that your *sister also died of* BC (one of
hundreds ... thousands ...

— River Styx —

... millions ...

(1) 'cigarette burn' port hole below the left neck (2) port
slash under left clavicle (3) left chest gash (flared, untidy)
(4) right chest (far —

— elevator, one short floor, exit to —

Shorn *Dwarf Siberian* kale recovers by increments.

Hazy ... hot ...

Disappearance of ducks on Reynolds Pond... normal
summer (?) —

— orange short-sleeved shirt from her —

We clipped one another's wrist bracelets when we came
home with scissors from the sewing cabinet.

— loose enough to camouflage the pair of fleshy nubs
('dog ears') on either side of the sternum —

(1) buy a cheap tennis racket (2) fail to call oncologist (3)
convince yourself that a parallel lumpiness —

— of value should I make it to April (two-year —

Fail, fail again —

— do they go in summer or some kind of field trip?

Fail better.

— such a charming documentary on 'birders' in Central Park that I want a pair of birdy binoculars should I reach another birthday, ten weeks —

— LEAST I'LL BE SYMMETRICAL —

Burgeoning desire to pack up, move to Manhattan and go 'birding' with this group of friendly bird-nerds.

NEVER HAVE TO BUY ANOTHER —

The expert leader is an older woman with terminal breast cancer who announces that she wants to experience as much as she can for as long as she can. She has eighty notebooks compiled over decades, accounts of every single bird —

IMPROVEMENT IN MY POSTURE —

Easily a hundred or more blackbirds from nowhere (beginning to shower, welcome before the next heat wave), having gotten wind that the small but thick, lush, cartoon-green, organic back lawn harbors microscopic gourmet vittles, squawk and stab away, fluttering among the cuke-zukes by the fence as reinforcements arrive, muddy brown souls among the blacks.

A neighbor peers over at the Hitchockian scene from her driveway.

— screen door sweep to the sky in a huff — neighboring oaks —

Those orange perennials are *day lilies.*

Up before six with the *quank—quank—quank* —

'Wild Suburban Kingdom' with Marlon Perkins?

Bartleby —

If —

Should I pick this lone *Jalapeño* before some salsa-loving critter snatches it?

— prefer not —

Ditto the *Boston Pickling?*

Opening Day, u-pick blueberries!

— prefer —

EVERYTHING PROGRESSING WELL.

Conservatively, the two of us picked some <u>nine hundred</u> pounds: fifteen pounds per visit (seven to eight pounds apiece), five or six annual excursions over fifteen years, fewer when I lived on the West Coast.

SURGEON AMAZED AT HER RAPID RECOVERY
AND HEALING.

My first (her wide-brimmed straw hat; her methodical picking; her bucket fuller than mine when we met up) solo outing.

Cool and dry morning.

SAID LIVER WAS —

Huge lovely berries.

I gather over seven pounds ($20.05) in my bucket and make a lattice-crusted blueberry —

... AS CAN BE EXPECTED, BUT NONETHELESS,
STILL STAGE —

— pint of glistening *Blueberry Sauce,* recipe in her distinct Catholic penmanship in the wooden box, bundled alphabetically in 'Miscellaneous' after *Blueberry Buckle, Blueberry Cobbler, Blueberry Crisp, Blueberry Fancy Crust, Blueberry Pudding* ...

Last summer we were too unwell to pick.

I did not imagine —

— <u>one thousand</u> pounds —

— IN TOWN TO LOOK OVER THE INVALIDS BUT
SHE'S FALLING INTO A COMA BECAUSE WE'RE
NOT MUCH FUN.

Mid-July heat index at 100°: (1) pull down shades
(2) attempt to push the contents of the ancient air
conditioned sunporch into the kitchen and den with the
help of four floor fans and two ceiling fans (3) shut
bathroom door, computer room door, her bedroom door
(4) first floor bearable, but leave windows cracked or
open depending on side of house, shade factor, etc.

Despite the sauna, an early morning trip to the sporting
goods store to investigate toddler baseball gloves.

— jaw —

A stop at the climate-controlled library, people flowing in
and flowing out —

— jaw, palpate the small —

Why everything so gendered (insufferable 'pinkiness')?

Call or not to —

— stroke —

    — palpate (regular appointment in two —

NB: My first glove over forty years ago was fire engine
red.

This is a wonderful gift to offer your loved one.

— stroke —

    — palpate —

— stroke —

    — one side—

— bullet train (illusion for a couple more weeks before slipping into 'active' —

... tests, scans, biopsies, appointments (living at the clinic—

The sacred Hour of Watering after dinner, puttering inch by inch through the garden, the herb patch, counting *Yellow* (green) *Pear* tomatoes —<u>thirteen</u> —

— *put you on blah blah* though you will very well —

— — anyway —

Dwee —

— and *blah blah* will not even —

Dwee-buh-dee —

Each pain-free — symptom-free —

    I LOVE YOU ALL.

To accept (a là Bette, kneeling and planting her —

— whole days and I do not think of —

ICD9: *197.7 Secondary Malig Neo Liver*

SUBJECT: HIGHLY UNPLEASANT NEWS

Blueberry tart is delicious.

How it is possible —

Another ant bomb detonates from a crack in the wall, swarming the defenseless *Boston Pickling*, butter blossoms (*eat me*), buried flag —

1. Sprinkle freebie Berbere seasoning (cayenne red pepper, garlic, ginger, fenugreek, cardamom, cumin, black pepper, allspice, turmeric, cloves, Ceylon cinnamon and coriander) on all leaves.
2. Spoon more 'Critter Ridder' around bases.

Freshly snipped *Genovese* basil and Greek oregano across my 'pizzapiece' —

3. Drop extra Predascent© capsules along stone borders.
4. Spritz more undiluted apple cider vinegar over the *(eat me)* dandelion meadow in the 'pool' ring (though 'chucks seem to enjoy this dressing on their greens).

Sturdy sprawl of *Black Beauty* zuke leaves against the house.

> 5. Sprinkle pepper seasoning (cayenne, garlic, paprika, red pepper flakes, bell peppers) on leaves and base.

The *Jalapeño* buds more fruit — five or six doll peppers.

> 6. Pour watering can of water over the ant mob — watch them swirl, regroup, carry on.

Elephantine leaves and yellow bell flowers flow onto the walkway.

I train the fuzzy *Boston Pickling* vine around the black railing post so the mailman won't stumble.

Where animals retreat in this heat?

... enough ...

> CAN'T HELP BUT FEEL I COULD BE FERRIED OFF
> AT ANY MINUTE WITH A RUPTURED SPLEEN —

— to find someone qualified to install two safety 'grab' bars along the bathtub walls, though she would only take two more —

... enough ...

In their fur coats?

— OR HEART ATTACK OR PULMONARY
EMBOLISM —

Long enough.

Seven hours I shall never have again, culling her
wasteland of medical bills —

Irregularities, mistakes, oversights.

— to get my kinky, permy hair cut, first foray in fifteen
months —

Ten or so of these 'events' into a clear orange plastic
folder for follow-up.

Lawn, day sixteen, is a patchwork of clover, mismatched
grasses, lamb's ear, dandelions, and moss by the lilac.
Still too hot to mow; heat index near $100°$.

LIKE I HAVE THE FLU …

Sneakers plow through grassy slush to snag my daily
arugula.

ENORMOUS, ENORMOUS FATIGUE.

— four days from now, at which time the grass may well
be seven, eight inches (?!) —

I'LL HAVE HAIR FOR ANOTHER TWO WEEKS.

— when I can pull out the mower and roll Zen row after
Zen —

— EVEN TO EAT RIGHT NOW. LIKE HAVING A
GARBAGE PAIL IN YOUR MOUTH ALL THE TIME.

I clip the inaccessible grass by the house, beneath the
hose, beside the walkway garden, on hands and knees on
the folded old bathmat with the retro manual clippers.
I work my way around the edging stones, three tomato
pots, the side of the stairs leading down to the driveway.

MY SKULL ACHES.

Neglected prairie grasses poke out beneath the hose rack
where water drips.

MY BONES HAVE THE FLU.

— burst, 9:33 AM — completion of call to clinic to have
my August 2nd appointment moved up to Tuesday, July
23, 3:30 PM; bloodwork, 3:15 PM.

... *swollen lymph node in my* —

First shiny, fat *Jalapeño* plucked and chopped fine onto
refried bean tacos. I remove ribs and seeds to tame, but
for many hours, even lying in bed that evening, my
fingers tingle.

— old e-files, miscellaneous flash drives, assorted —

Tan Bunny twitches in the clover, ignoring the stunted,
shit-spattered blossoms.

— magnificent yellow zuke —

— pity on the parched sparrows, I mist the maple with several hose passes.

The cuke vine along the top of the staircase has shot out a good two —

Grateful *dwee-buh-dee — dwee —*

Several more *Black* (green) *Krim* tomatoes and some three dozen *Yellow* (green) *Pears.*

Last of the shaker of 'Triple Kelp Seaweed' mulched along the base of each.

Even if — *sera* —

What Van Gogh would — with such Yellowness —

— *sera* —

> ... PREVIEW OF DYING, WHICH IS WHY I THINK
> IT'S NOT HARD TO MAKE —

— to type, and time —

— backward, not forward —

Key Largo, surprisingly good— such a cast!

— combination of fans, shades, ancient AC in the sunporch —

What do I —

What I do —

— mass on the — no mass —-

— left —

    — right —

— left —

    — right —

— left —

— *sera* —

— mass on the —

— glob of (glorious day lilies beam beneath the hottest —

    — TO DROP THINGS, A SMALL DISH OF SYRUP
    THIS MORNING ON THE FLOOR.

Tower of boxes:

A few wiry white hairs embedded in the back of the
maroon flowered rocker.

— ephemera; jottings; old reading notebook —

Time passes.
That is all.
SAMUEL BECKETT

— some fifteen years of —

— last lines written for the stage.)

Inexcusable to travel, or even live, without
taking notes.
FRANZ KAFKA

— breaks, barely, enough to attend the overgrown —

UPSETTING AS YOU CAN —

DISORIENTATION (time, place identity)

Less than 48 hours to the —

BREATHING PATTERN CHANGE

— struggle to push through row after row of damp
green—

This is called Cheynes-Stokes breathing.

He suggests more 'gland' than 'node' —

This may indicate readiness for the final —

NEW REALITY —

CT scan of the neck, Friday morning.

— GAPING —

How we could have —

> *I know I must go on doing this dance on hot
> bricks until I die.*
> VIRGINIA WOOLF

5:10 AM alarm: coffee, juice, a slice of my oatmeal-rosemary-raisin toast the three requisite hours before the contrast—

ICD9: 198.2 Secondary Malig Neo Skin

— warm clinic towel and repeated 'pings' to my left arm in an attempt to mine —

(Bette, kneeling and planting —

*"HOW IS THE PEACH FUZZ ON YOUR HEAD? ARE
YOU FEELING A LITTLE —"*

ICD9: 197.7 Secondary Malig Neo Liver

"I HAPPEN TO LIKE THE LOOK OF SINEAD —"

... (contrast dye) warmth through the groin ... *breathe* ...
wind ... moors ... *breathe* ... heather ...

Hold your breath.

... heather ... moors ...

Do not swallow.

... wind ... *breathe* ... heather (Bette —

(Bette —

... wind ... *breathe* ...

Breathe.

Breathe.

No.

... wind ...

No.

No.

<u>Not</u> lymph node.

Asymmetrical salivary gland?

— of no clinical ? —

Hold your loved one's—

— glob of cancer is not a glob of —

Speak gently.

— two big bunches of *Lemon Thai* basil, toasted almonds, garlic, lemon juice, salt, pepper —

UNUSUAL COMMUNICATION: Accept the moment as a beautiful gift.

Is anyone —

— pesto linguini with steamed zucchini and sun-dried —

Baby W, or Adolescent W, having doubled or trebled his or her body weight, is on the scene again, nibbling clover in the Magic Pool Ring and nosing around the neighbor's flower beds.

I dole out more coyote pellets along the wall and fence, and garlic powder in a wavery line along the walkway border.

Tan Bunny nibbles clover in the Magic Pool Ring.

Bees nudge the *Jalapeños*, seven stout green fruit.

AUGUST

"How the mud goes round in the mind —
what a swirl these monsters leave ..."

VIRGINIA WOOLF, "AN UNWRITTEN NOVEL"

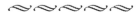

Forty, fifty *Yellow* (green) *Pear* tomatoes on the vine!
Four handsome *Black* (green) *Krim* tomatoes in the clay
pot.

I position the hose on its side in the grass, nozzle pointed
in the direction of potential critters to mimic a
'scaresnake'.

First Resurrection in several weeks.

The geraniums have been removed.

Heat wave grasses yellow the plot.

Dried leaves dot the ground and road from some of the
trees, autumnal harbinger, though the temperature
soars—

Dud Reckoning: all carrots, the *Flat of Italy* onions, every cuke and zuke along the lilac fence (sun-blocking maple canopy —

Cortical lichen —

On the physical level, the body begins the final process —

(blocks of ice when I rolled down the compression —

> THANKS SO MUCH FOR THE ZA'ATAR. EXTRA
> COOL COMING FROM JERUSALEM.

— fatigue and indolence; waves of summer visitors.

> HOPE TO CRACK INTO IT SOON IF AND WHEN I
> GET SOME TASTE BUDS.

White powdery mildew (?) spots coat the *Black Beauty* zuke leaves.

Male blossoms explode early morning, then shrivel back into themselves.

Females continue MIA.

Since mid-summer heat wave, garden growth arrested.

Overwatered?

This is — ?

Gone dormant?

Black Krim: five handsome green-orange tomatoes.
One for lunch, sun-warm, dripping down my chin.

Normal?

Sweet, juicy *Yellow Pear* snack, half dozen plus daily.

Several fat-crisp *Boston Pickling* cukes from the staircase
vine and the wall vine.

(Prickles deter critters?)

Pale yellow *Santa Fe* peppers, like wax beans.

Doll-sized green *Serrano Tampiqueno* on the tall plant by
the wall.

Single vine twisting through the fence, one stunted cuke
along the rail, poking through the neighbor's yard.

Bee magnet *Thai* basil — bushy purple flowers.

Lemon basil past prime.

Genovese basil squat but enough for salad, sandwiches,
pizza.

Mr. or Ms. W emerges for another bow, well fattened for
the coming winter, and plows through the freshly
mowed smorgasbord of grass, clover, moss, dandelions,
and lambs ear, ignoring, again, the garden beneath the
wall.

Tan Bunny AWOL.

— eyes fixed on a certain spot, no blinking —

I creep to the wall, hover a foot away, and give a small shout.

Puppet turns and waddles, greens-stuffed, along the top of the wall, west then south back to the cemetery, planting himself near the summer-abandoned burrow.

Bee waltz: bud — basil — bud —

Fragrant basil flowers.

Cilantro gone fast to white flower, belying the *Slo-Bolt* label but enough for a pinch in the salsa with one of the crunchy fresh *Jalapeños* (even deveined and deseeded, the party in the back yard coughs over their chips).

Cukes in the grass tripling (!) — fourpling (!) in size overnight —

I do uproot the dud *Black Beauty* zuke beside the house before noticing a single pollinated baby zucchini – first and only of the summer.

(Murderer.)

I strip the dead yellow mildewed leaves off the more salvageable specimen, drop it back in the ground, and tamp the roots.

Leaves and stems twitch and wither like the witch's feet in Oz.

Disappearance of walk and wall chipmunks.

Occasional lean squirrel on a flagstone.

Robins snap worms.

Gangs of chickadees (wrens?) descend, plotting mischief.

Lo, in the morning, a new green shoot and leaf, and a yellow male blossom reopens, expectant.

Where oh where are the *female* —

Origin of that dark palm-sized poop in the lower yard, abuzz with flies — ?

An invasive weed shoots above the wall, crazy rapid growth between the sad zucchini and the pale kale. I prune to wall height. Pods form. Many green berries.

Kale too bitter (heat wave?). Replant at the far corner beside the spent day lilies, eye toward autumn —

Pokeweed, I am informed.

— over a month between mowings now — arrested —

'Eau–de-Cut-Grass' ...

A quarter mile down the road, church bells (carrot duds; red onion duds —

New Haven mantel clock, then the Elgin Westminster.

Eleven —

The Anti-Calendar: my sister's — *nine years* on Tuesday (lightning split the tree in the yard beneath the window—

— in formation up over the neighbors' roof, flying fast, heading to —

Replanted spinach, lettuce, kale seeds set upon by gangs of thuggy robins.

SEPTEMBER

"A higher truth, though only dimly hinted at,
thrills us more than a lower expressed."

HENRY DAVID THOREAU, JOURNAL

Cotton clouds at ludicrous altitude (-70° out the window)

— no sensation *she is here* —

— *anywhere* —

Cold mist across the Avenues, the wide, familiar
sidewalks, tricking motion detector lights on pale pastel
houses.

— *somewhere* —

Blue as ever — the Pacific —

I MISS HER EVERY DAY.

Yes, the sky; hypnotic orange Bridge unchanged —

On what would have been her 80th, pictures emailed
around the country: (1) Pink Red Sox cap, sunglasses.
Blue sky and beach, big smile. (2) Almost giddy,
enjoying a cup of her favorite maple walnut ice cream on
a bench beside —

> *"AS DO I."*
> *"WE ALL DO."*

I revisit the de Young Museum and drift among —

> *"I DO, TOO."*

— so tired of saying *I'm so* —

Tired, tired —

Tears express your love and help you to let go.

At the top of China Beach in my old neighborhood I am
too tired to broach either the descent to the beach itself —
twist of concrete road or steep strip of stairs embedded in
the hillside (one must, like Ginger Rogers, *go back — up—*

> OPERATED ON AS I WRITE TO HAVE A HIP
> REPLACEMENT.

Fine vistas nonetheless of Bridge and water and boats —

I snag the lone wooden bench as soon as it is vacated.
How often I'd strolled down to the sand, this shore —

> CRASHED TO THE FLOOR, COULDN'T—

The same occurred at Land's End, forced to retreat halfway when confronted with startling staircases.

Creak of bones, brain and knees.

Skipping — ragged heart —

Horseflies alight on my bare arms, impossible to flick away.

Circle and return, circle and —

RESTLESSNESS (repetitive motions such as —

Driven from the bench (— Fly buzz — when I —

>*Maybe* —

Blue-gray waves (how we could have —

Nine years. I came back to her hospice, her second floor bedroom. We chatted about my vacation. I said I ate and drank to excess.

COME UP SOONER RATHER THAN —

She said *that's what vacations are for.*

Bougainvillea climbs the houses.

She was hard to make out, her voice was so —

My pair of cat charges, Fiona and Princess Igor, loll on
the ground, agitated by the appearance of sun.

Hours of lolling, barely moving, until Princess stretches
— yawns — makes her way to the stockade fence — and
leaps to the top in one pounce, from which vantage she
patrols, back arched, on her Hot Tin —

GETTING READY TO GO TO THE REHAB 'GYM'.

Back and forth, balance beam —

WORKING ON HER UPPER ARM STRENGTH,
SOME STAIRS, SHOE TYING ...

This is called Cheynes-Stokes breathing.

— into the neighbor's yard for several hours.

Repeat. Repeat. Repeat. Repeat.

Repeat.

— TOO FAR OFF THOUGH I CANNOT SAY FOR —

Repeat.

A fog mass obscures the feeble sun; impossible to tell
time of day or even —

On my third full day in town, my flippy chemo-do becomes insufferable in the Pacific breezes, so I walk twenty blocks west towards Ocean beach to a tiny Asian budget salon, researched online to the best of my instincts.

Repeat.

I explain to the middle-aged, agreeably hip stylist that (1) I've lost all my hair to chemotherapy (2) I've not had a haircut in eighteen months (3) my head has morphed into a factory of unwelcome perm-curls (4) her mission is to chop off as many of the *Annie* curls as possible and topiary the remainder into something semi-palatable.

(No repercussions from the flying, despite ignoring the suggestion to be fitted for a prophylactic —

I revisit the de Young —

Fifteen minutes, much raucous (Chinese?) hilarity with her compatriot snipping away at the next chair, and twenty-three dollars later, I nod my startled approval to the mirror.

> ❖ *Chariot of Death Carrying the Angel of Death.*
> (cottonwood, horsehair, marbles, leather,
> paper, fabric, paint, ca. 1900)

Sometimes there's *god — so quickly* ...

Changes: everyone (except me and one older gent) on the trolley plugged into some small, crack-like device —

—*anywhere* —

— cafés, the Bridge, the old —

A cool, moist washcloth on the forehead may increase physical comfort.

> ❖ <u>*Coffin in the shape of a cocoa pod*</u> (wood, paint, cloth, ca 1970).

DECREASED SOCIALIZATION: If you are part of the final inner circle of support, the person needs your affirmation, support, and —

— *quank—quank* high up in the —

— *nowhere* —

OCTOBER

"Tomorrow and tomorrow and tomorrow..."

WILLIAM SHAKESPEARE, MACBETH

Bushy brown and black caterpillars slither across my
path.

— even drought-bound cannot help but go on, though
Slo-Bolt long bolted, now 'coriander' —

Beige strongbox: laminated birth certificates; wedding
certificate; mortgage papers —

 Vigil for the abrupt rupture, summer to fall (death of
short-sleeves; unsecured lawn chairs; screen windows
and doors), though today's temperature —

Showers pelt the house, scattering russet, orange, red
maple leaves to the ground to dry in crisp, seductive
piles.

Pumpkin porches —

Cornstalks strangle mailboxes and lightposts.

Wind, winds, beginning bareness on the upper, outer branches —

PHYSICAL SIGNS: an orderly progression of physical changes

Despite the drought and heat wave in my three-week absence: three dozen *Yellow Pear* and two *Black Krim* on the —

— one plump red and two green bell peppers —

Basil —

— neon orange *Santa Fe* pepper —

Giant of Italy parsley shoots up after the rain.

Thai and lemon basil flowers —

You may help your loved one by giving permission to let —

Cukes and zukes dead — dried — curled against the ground.

Slender, ornamental *Serranos* on the sole surviving plant.

Dwarf Siberian kale curly leaves, enough —

— affirm the individual's ongoing value —

— indefatigable rosemary; oregano; thyme —

Squirrels streak the yard — urgent —

— good you will carry forward —

Premature hibernation? 'chucks, Tan Bunny, robins, jays, cardinals, chipmunks —

More leaves on the road along the golfy turf, and the birches now shedding.

Never assume the person <u>cannot hear.</u>

Lord, lord, I've killed a fine specimen of spider sidling across the blue bedspread, crumpled Kleenex mashed against the wooden floor. (Yes, *Charlotte's Web*, but two raised welts — bites? — along my waistline. Def *not* mosquito —

6:30 PM, nearly dark.

'lesions' redder (beginnings) than yesterday ... ?

> ... COTTON SWAB METHOD TONIGHT, NUMBING UP THE TARGET AREAS TO THE BEST OF MY ABILITY AND EATING IMMEDIATELY, AS SOON AS IT FELT NUMBED —

Bites?

> BETTER, ALLOWING ME TO GET THROUGH THE MEAL WITHOUT EXCRUCIATING —

White butterfly among the pale purple *Thai* flowers.

How much longer (lifespan of the common —

— shoulder blade; folded the washcloth over and over for a clear, blood-free square; blotted gently.

AGAIN AT THE POINT OF STOPPING —

Rubbed antibacterial ointment across the bloody, oozing scab.

Large square bandage over everything.

— uncommon —

Helped guide arms into sleeves, head into hole.

Reassured her that it did, indeed, look better, that it was, in fact (immaterial), less —

— *better* than the day —

— getting *better* —

— looking —

— whole days —

Tower of boxes:

— crusted gauze from the sticky, oozing scab.

Blotted, blotted ...

— photos; letters; tchotchkes (my Shakespeare shot glass
from Stratford-upon-Avon); clippings; yearbooks;
personalized pencils (?) —

47° and the pair of *Black Krims* hold fast (first reluctant
turn of thermostat) —

— until a blister forms in the crack of my left thumb,
friction between metal pole and blue cloth glove.

Mini mountains of brown, red, and orange leaves across
the yard, packed into three tall paper lawn bags for
collection.

— *better* —

About 95% of foliage remains on the maple and assorted
cemetery trees overhanging the yard; conservative
estimate: another sixty bags required?

Manic post-rake squirrel action, winter food foraging —

Whole days without a single —

Leaves crumble and compact, layer upon layer beneath
my gloved hands.

— *better* —

Each tall bag swallows many more piles than anticipated, and the yard looks remarkably tidier after a good hour.

Still the outline, disparity between turf and reseeded plot eight months on.

How long before the seamless blend into brethren *Laroche, Dubois, Dussault, Ouellette, Hetu, Leger, Bouchard, Brissart* ...

WWI block: Doughboys & Wives.

When I inquired about eco-caskets the facilitator demurred. My mother clutched her purse as we shuffled from room to room through the casket 'showcase'.

Her cedar box atop my father's pine box atop —

Cheap caskets designed as ugly as possible (Fred Flintstone bathtub?) to nudge the bereaved to upgrade. She, the most discriminating of shoppers, found something midrange, a shiny pine she was sure that he, the most particular of men, would have approved.

GIVING PERMISSION:

The closed casket disappointed some, no doubt.

Your ability to give assurance that it is all right to let go is one of the greatest —

Yellow polo shirt, gray sweatpants, underwear and socks in a plastic bag.

I don't know why he needs socks, she said.

We shrugged and smiled.

As it is near 70°, I revisit Ancient Green Pitchfork Implement (rusted; rounded; sharp-tined) to step on its shoulders and hack a square around the 'pokeweed', which has become 'pokemonster', more tree than weed, with a wide fat trunk, and roots many fathoms —

Tugging with all my unimpressive strength budges —

— passes and hacks, deep gouges through the wall soil before snapping through at least part of the root formation, a whitish bulb the size of a potato (?).
I lift what I can of the fat pokeweed and her smaller sibling, wary of what I might leave — 'Johnny Pokeweed'—

Withered cukes and zukes, vines coiled into the refuse pile.

Snip another orange-red *Santa Fe* —

For variation, I walk the river. Though the foliage is not yet peak, the colors are lovely; paths leaf-strewn; squirrels busy; currents frothing; dam scenic; bikers courteous.

Along the fence some of the rail posts have been removed from their sockets and flung overboard, where they now rise out of the muck below, detritus among the grasses, moss, algae, underbrush.

Gaps like broken teeth.

A pair of birders, clutching binoculars, tell me they are stalking 'herons'!

First sighting of Canadian geese at Resurrection — eight or nine puttering on the grass.

Sightings: brown baby *frog* in the garden, first I've seen since childhood.

Slug on one of the last surviving cukes (first encounter with a slug outside 'Ramona' —

So many leaves on the lawn.

Beginning of the end for the *Boston Picklings*, leaves turning yellow and brown. Some fruit grows oddly — bulbous — while others perfect on the same vine.

Dwarf Siberian holds on salads —

Three dozen *Yellow* (green) *Pears* — second crop — since September.

Wall kale demolished by 'grasshoppers' according to my—

Crisp, spiny exteriors, soft explosion of seeds in the —

Coming attraction: goose poop in random decoration
along the circular —

— flotilla of pocketbooks (enough to open a consignment
shop); toothbrushes; travel containers —

> — PARTIALLY COLLAPSED LUNG AND HAD TO BE
> HOSPITALIZED OVERNIGHT —

— page after page of 'proxy' financial documents, within
seconds of my arrival in the crowded, hot, institutional—

> SECOND ATTEMPT SUCCESSFUL.

Outside her room, unending cackling. The 'inmate' doors
were not permitted *(No Exit)* to be —

> SHE HAD TO HAVE HER FAULTY PORT REMOVED
> AND REDONE —

The admitting doctor squatted beside the vinyl easy chair
and suggested that the solution to her current
predicament was to *eat some Dorritos.*

'chuck edges the garden but opts for her preferred clover.

> WE ARE BOTH ABOUT READY TO DIG UP JACK
> KEVORKIAN.

Port, forty-eight hours —

Gumcracker denied that the open venous line, taped to her chest and 'overlooked' at time of ER discharge, was in any way —

ICD9: 174.9 Malign Neopl Breast NOS (Primary)

— circle of oldsters as one male patient performed his Tai Chi-ish exercises.

> GENUINE 5:00 BABY FLUFF SHADOW ON MY SKULL.

— decibel-bending, protracted, slow motion ('mouse'?!!

I caught her eye from the doorway to extricate her from this activity. We returned partway with the walker, but she had to finish the journey in her wheelchair.

Obituaries for women under 60 are almost all, by default—

I argued up the skill level food chain until it was agreed that the line *should be* —

> — SAYS I'M LIKE SINEAD O'CONNOR (MYSTERIOUSLY HIPLY).

Observation: when a body can no longer support standing weight —

We talked about my vacation.

— sister, father, mother —

I helped her to the bathroom, bare squeak of voice, trying
to instruct me how to support her beneath the armpits
(her young children sequestered downstairs).

— **affirm the individual's ongoing value to you and the good
you will** —

I waited outside the door for a long while, then knocked
and went in to help her rise, as she could not —

Russet leaves brighten in ever greater numbers, tumbling
over the just-raked yard.

Balm of morning black and chill New England —

— pair of *Black* (pale green) *Krims* —

Tufts of parsley, rosemary, oregano, thyme —

Weeks and nary a mention —

— nothing —

On the radio, advertisements for funeral parlors and
home health services, *your time of need* —

Pale sky —

A hornet claws, claws the screen —

Lower branches dance —

Bare twigs up high — what is coming —

Where do they go?

— she go —

— he go —

When two middle school boys sail through the Resurrection gates, plotting skateboard acrobatics, I hesitate before approaching.

— they go —

You have to think of people coming to visit loved ones.

— walkers, mostly singletons, one or two without fail —

Water the *Black Krims* in the still bright sunshine.

(They do retreat.)

The geezer who parks in the far right turnoff, swings a golf club at the horizon, wags his plumber's ass crack —

Beige (unlocked, keyless) strongbox in the back of her closet: legal envelopes; records; papers; cemetery deeds...

Grave location: Sec 3, Lot —

Mémère's death certificate, IMMEDIATE CAUSE (find condition resulting in death): ACUTE CEREBROVASCULAR ACCIDENT

In 1982, 'Nine Hundred and Ninety Dollars for the right of interment in Perpetual Care 3 Grave, Lot. No. — Section — of Resurrection Cemetery.'

Pépère's death certificate: PROSTATE CANCER

Monument, Caron Granite Company, $821.50.

A pale blue pamphlet, *Rules and Regulations for Catholic Diocesan Cemeteries, Providence, June 1ˢᵗ, 1980:*

Under <u>Notes </u>on the last blank page Pépère (presumably) had penciled in the dimensions: 3'6" wide, underlined twice (size limit for monument —

> *"Idling, loafing, loitering or any boisterous demonstration within the Cemetery is prohibited."*

Church records: my mother's colorful, pictorial 'Souvenir de baptième' twelve days after her birth in 'Ste. Anne, par le Rev. A.O. Fournier'.

— THIS MORNING AT 7:30, PEACEFULLY.

'Remembrance of first holy Communion in St. Matthew's Church', age 6 —

BE WELL.

'Souvenir de Confirmation', age 11, 'dans l'eglise de Saint Joseph le 29 avril 1945'.

Papers for my father's service: Merchandise: Pine Tree Casket, $2,800.

Earlier dusk encroaches, 6:00 PM.

Total: $10,678.

Bushels of leaves, like the loaves and the fish, replenish the raked lawn.

Halloween in the air.

Small pumpkins on some graves.

Leaves do, literally, 'crackle'.

Piles, piles of leaves.

Worrisome digestion (indigestion) plus sluggish bowels plus bloating —

Trawling, trawling (ovarian *blah blah*) to the point of (*blah blah blah* —

Should we call this — interstice — 'the gloaming'.

Crisp mornings, brisk and breezy jacket afternoons.

... papers; pamphlets; folders; forms ...

I LOVE YOU ALL.

— soon, could well be —

Punctured (refrigerator; cars grinding down the main —

**— preparation for release, a detaching from surroundings
and relationships —**

Elgin and New Haven clocks prepare to —

— unresponsive, withdrawn, or in a comatose-like state.

Remove t-shirts. Transfer sweaters and long-sleeved —

— foggy wide avenues straight down to the Pacific —

After lapses, fresh purges.

Top drawer: plastic 'Pietà' *Vatican Pavilion, New York
World's Fair, 1964-5*, which may have been purchased as a
souvenir, or for the babysitting Mémère and Pépère.

Dad's death certificate: LYMPHOMA

The youngest were not included in this curious
expedition, though I believe I attended in utero.

How many decks of *Bicycle* playing cards, opened and
unopened —

Mom's death certificate: BREAST CANCER, STAGE IV

File folder of extended family obituaries, clippings, funeral cards: Mémère's, Pépère's, my sister's, father's, now my mother's from the local —

— THIS MORNING AT 7:30, PEACEFULLY.

— these contraptions, items in the 'Broken Hip Kit' she was made to purchase last January.

Chunky plastic yellow blade, looped with a thick cord for *putting on socks.* Cheap sponge on a stick for *washing toes.* Her favorite, the arm-extending pincher known as the 'Reacher' for *picking things off the* —

— *chang* — walker on wooden — *chang* —

— walker on linoleum —

— *chang-chang* —

Sluggish bowels (abated).

Yes — to monitor —

Belly bites (faded).

Mystery cheek zit?

— *chang* —

— migraine that forced me to lie on the —

Several black garbage bags of clothes, shoes, coats have been taken to *Goodwill* and the *Savers* store at the plaza.

Dry cough (humidity)? Lack of —

　　　　Maybe —

Good, if dated, wardrobe.

A few pieces are my sister's, taken years ago after —

Fall cleanup: flush hose; turn off corresponding valve in the basement.

Giant yellow shoehorn. (Note: all these implements a 'cheerful' yellow.)

— gaping expanse of driveway, post-Honda sale —

Cheap wooden pole with metal prongs, the function of which eludes me. *Shoe-tying?*

Pinpoint clavicle sting (burn)?

Cords of Ziplocked blueberries, quart bags in gallon bags, stacked in the freezer.

How many — so many —

For the service I wrote a blueberry-themed remembrance.

Halfway through, a violent tear-trigger rose in my throat, but I was able to pause, compose and conclude without—

— INTO THE QUE SERA, SERA —

Silence in the interval; everyone watching my tightrope—

Crisp leaves embed themselves in the basil, oregano, pepper stalks, kale shoots —

Crisp leaves along the cemetery wall; trees flush —

Madcap *quank-quank,* maple and forsythia —

That bags of leaves are so quantifiable appeals.

— not mole — *growth* —

(The coincidence of the tree-splitting lightning so soon afterward astonished everyone.)

Whisper of clouds crosses the full moon.

Better, much better —

New Haven clock chimes *seven — eight — nine —* followed by the —

Overcast, but one of the last days to pick at peak foliage, so I head thirty miles north to my favorite orchard. Midweek, I am the sole customer.

Half-bushel bag in hand, I pick my way up the hillside overlooking forest and road; palette of gold, bronze, copper ...

Wooden signs nailed to trees at the ends of rows indicate variety: *Cortland, Mutsu, Gala, Macoun, Jonagold, Macintosh—*

Hundreds, maybe thousands on the ground in every permutation: cores — rotted — perfect — rotting.

Never assume the person <u>cannot</u> —

In fifteen minutes I fill my bag with *Macouns*, by size for eating, about the circumference of my small palm.

 Speak gently.

I balance a few wildcard *Mutsus* and *Cortlands* on top of the quivering bag.

Eyes on the skies, chipmunks tunnel ferociously through cemetery underbrush, broken branches, matted leaves —

— *Paula Red, Honey Crisp* —

Rotting apples and rotting —

I fill four more paper lawn bags to the brim, tamp down with my gloves and fold the tops over neatly, flurries to the coming blizzard.

Delicious decay and damp.

Woods in the nostrils.

Insomnia radio smothers my whirring —

Tired, so tired —

USE 4 DROPS SUBLINGUALLY EVERY 4 HOURS

Decomposition (a few weeks ago, Pacific on the breeze; homeless on the trolley —

An unusual lapse in medical bills, hers <u>and</u> mine.

Tired, so —

Have we been forsaken?

A year ago, the mouse behind her chair, down some crack in the wall.

I set cheap wooden traps with dabs of peanut butter beside the furnace.

Millions of leaves in bags from (a) the maple (b) nameless cemetery trees overhanging the wall.

We caught one, then two — four in all — and dumped the traps (shocked eyes open —

Identify by 'leaf structure'?

— brown trash barrel (thus the scream from the kitchen—

— my first —

> *Does the tree bear cones and have leaves that are needle-like?*
> *Does the tree have leaves that are flat and thin and shed annually?*

Not too late to walk in the overcast, cool, leaf-strewn —

> *Are the leaves PINNATELY COMPOUND, blades with deeply toothed or LOBED MARGINS?*

Front lawn sere.

Leafmania.

Cigarette butts; paper cups; plastic bottles; and torn candy wrappers dot sidewalk and driveway edges.

— tying of shoes at a distance?

Sisyphean gloved plucking —

Beyond delirious, I took the laptop into bed with me, 4:30ish AM, to pound out a two-page single-spaced update of her condition to fax to her oncologist, Dr. N—, before the morning's readmittance.

Where have the 'chucks — Tan Bunny —

— wherefore art —

— *much better* —

Chipmunks mobilize through the —

Flirtation with 70°; garden flummoxed: *aren't we dying,*
say the *Thai* basil, the lemon basil —

What time it is —

— *Yellow Pear* tomatoes, clusters of green babes a-
popping —

Two white flowers on the *Jalapeño* (?)

Bumblebee pinballs among the purple basil blossoms,
though distinct yellowing, a hardening to the main stalk
on the biggest tomato plant.

Last two *Black Krim* on the windowsill to ripen.

A few kale leaves by the house for lunch.

What to do with the dozen dangling *Serranos,* when even
the *Jalapeños* blew roofs off mouths.

Enough, enough —

One gone yellow — too far gone —

— through the cyberswamp for information: *Compassion & Choices*

— aren't we —

Call I would make to one of the — might make —

— am I (left jawline; one finger, two fingers — noticeable absence on the —

— sluggish bowels —

End of Life Consultation: We Can Help —

EVERY 4 HOURS AS NEEDED

"... achieve a peaceful death —"

Two delirious single-spaced pages (half an hour to configure fax, laptop and landline —

— mice from slipping through —

Hello.

— leaf-blower noise pollution —

— could well be —

I did suggest, breaking down, that if she refused food and water she could slip into a —

I need some information.

— (weeping even as I —

— no blinking —

— when the time — that she had — 'some control'—

— jaw relaxed and mouth slightly —

Branches jangle; gold and orange leaves in the sun.

Post-raking, substantial piles matted in the fences, at the base of the trunk, spread out across the lawn in drifts and pools.

Trees wave in the woods behind the neighbors' –

Property shaggier than any time in the last fifty years of occupation.

— eyes fixed on a certain spot —

Long grasses mat against the chain-link fence and curl around the fire hydrant on the front lawn.

Weed tufts poke out of cracked walls and driveway.

Random leaves accumulate on the stairs, beside the shed, around the trash barrels.

Alarming pieces of roof flake onto the lawn.

The northern, sunless side of the house against the cemetery coated in a green, algae-like film.

Safe in their Alabaster Chambers — none of the four would approve —

> *Untouched by Morning —*
> *And untouched by noon —*

— but perhaps — understand —

Fr. R— swung by to perform last rites, or technically, the 'sacrament of the sick'.

— *blah blah*, recovering from total left hip ('Fax sent successfully') *blah blah* —

As she was no longer conscious, he barked prayers loudly into her ear, as if to raise her up like Lazarus from the loaner hospital bed.

How many times he must have —

Pinkitude – pinkiness (and here I wear a pink knit cap —

Four years prior he'd done a more muted variation for my father in the institutional hospice.

> *Grand go the Years — in the Crescent — above*
> *them —*

One of the attendants inquired in the foyer —

— tubing from around her head against the pillow, but—

Did you write that —

The silenced oxygen machine mirrored the stopped —

EVERY 4 HOURS AS NEEDED

We huddled in the chilly sunporch with the door closed while the funeral men, racing the coming blizzard, carried her down the front steps to the waiting —

— rackety *clatter*, effortful scraping and maneuvering of metal wheels on wooden stairs, stretcher and attendants that took my sister's body away.

Missing in action?

Then, too, I closed the family room door to shield her children —

— many days — whole chunks —

The kitchen clock is ill, first three or four *bongs*, more like *twangs* on a guitar out of —

Through the window, I survey the shriveled stalks of the finally dead tomatoes.

Thai basil, too, except for one patch sheltered by the purple flowers and heat-retaining concrete.

My toddler niece picks the last dozen *Yellow Pears*,
adding them to their siblings, in varying degrees of
ripeness, in the flat kitchen basket.

Twenty or so licorice leaves from these stalks.

An overnight leafstorm blankets the tidy yard, the dried
yellow grasses.

Nature's 'potato chips', addictive crackle and snuff —

Light frost coats the car windows and glazes the grass.

The furnace chugs on duty for the next six —

Rosemary undaunted.

Oregano and thyme carry on.

She said *I remember Nana*, as we flipped through the
photo calendar on the couch.

Pumpkins on so many —

Nana's gone to heaven.

High-wire squirrels along the chain-link —

Chipmunks in and out of wall cracks —

Blue jays from the cemetery forage the agitated, newly
raked yard.

Half, if not two-thirds remain, greeny-gold and russet,
ankle-deep —

Twitch — pain — spasm in the right —

— *sera* — *sera* —

A 'lasagna'-ish compost lark along the fence beneath the
lilac: dried chile stalks, cuke vines, basil flowers, mint
remains, brown and yellow tomato vines, soil contents of
the tomato buckets.

Add layers of leaves?

(I read and ignore the suggestion that they be 'shredded'
and watered.)

Add snow and wait?

— *dwee-buh-dee* fainter, fainter —

Another spring.

— *sera* — *sera* —

At the edges of Reynolds Pond, the black duck
contemplates the coming —

Cornstalks — lightposts —

The best strategy is calling directly (shower of fat, repetitive, premature holiday catalogues) — *my Mom passed away, please remove her* —

Another —

> *"... cordially invites you to join us as we*
> *remember your loved one at our Annual*
> *Memorial Mass for those who were buried*
> *in our parish from —"*

— Resurrection? After the tease (past the wrought iron entry gates: PLEASE ABSOLUTELY NO FEEDING THE GEESE! —

> *"... once the name of your loved one is read*
> *aloud, one of your family members are*
> *invited to come forward and place a —"*

Sleeping more frequently will occur with or without —

Three bags, four bags full —

A praying mantis (!) sidles along the concrete.

> *"... all who have passed on may enter the*
> *dwelling place that the Lord —"*

Evolution from <u>stare</u> (if male, default <u>ogle</u>) to <u>rapid glance away</u> —

Ripping roots, brown tomato plants in my gloved —

Puffs of leaf dust — compacted mass in brown paper —

Dad's fourth today — *four year* (bedside, his heavy hand—

(Bedside, her gnarled knuckles —

Bathroom shelves nine months on: Ziploc of wide square bandages; two tubes of 'mouth moisturizer' from the hospice team; bag of small blue sponges on sticks to cleanse the mouth —

Her leather address book with an insert of two folded sheets in Mémère's neat handwriting: birthdays of all children; grandchildren; great-grandchildren —

The last *Black Krim* blushes on the sill.

... eight packs of Bicycle playing cards, opened and unopened, some designated 'canasta'; pads of paper with grandchildren's pitch scores spanning many years —

Barish twigs through the maple top —

The pale yellow *Santa Fe* chile by the wall refuses —

I bake an appleberry pie with fruit I picked at three farms in two states: July blueberries (MA); August raspberries (NH); October apples (MA). I had not made this pie since February —

— *sera* — *sera* —

— (few — *yum* — bites before laying down the assistive—

On the radio, ads for funeral parlors and dementia care units, *if you or your loved one* —

A woman describes her parents urging her as a child to "look at every sunset as though it might be —"

— either side, tucked in pockets lined in the mastectomy camisole I was given at time of discharge.

Water as sewage. 'Platonic' municipal —

Once a day I unscrewed the rubber bulbs, dumped the accumulated pinkish chunky fluids into a plastic beaker, and recorded the amount, as per instructions, on a chart kept on the back of the —

Pink Cup, Blue Cup (colored straws in the clown box —

Gape of driveway — windblown leaves by the wall, beneath the shedding forsythia.

I REGRET, FOREMOST, THE LOSS OF MY —

I overturn a terracotta flower pot on the cement against the potential mousehole ('chuck-hole, critter-hole) at the base of the shed door.

This is a wonderful gift —

All he (or she, or they) wanted, ultimately, was the clover, of which there was an abundance in the upstairs yard where the ring of our childhood swimming pool once stood, and a patch beneath the lilacs, near the failed, too shady strip along the fence.

Horsefly between screen and —

Remove the plastic dressing or paper tape and gauze two days after your surgery.

Three boxelders sun themselves on the kitchen screen, cusp of November —

Leave the white steri-strips in place.

Bony bark, like hands or pitchforks against the sky.

They will fall off on their own.

— seasonal shutting of windows, muting the grinding cars —

The breast tissue has been sewn together and will heal.

Boo-wee — boo-wee — boo-wee — quank-quank —

The stitches dissolve and do not need to be removed.

Brown and white ducks —

Do not worry if the steri-strips fall off.

Air conditioner rocked gently from sill to floor.

Garden hose valve in basement.

Your wound will not open.

Rebecca Solnit's *The Faraway Nearby* crowns the precarious stack:

> *"I know how compelling ... stories are ...*
> *The teller goes in circles like a camel*
> *harnessed to a rotary water pump ..."*

Close the two spare rooms (her room).

> *"Feelings are kept alive that would fade*
> *away without narrative or are invented by*
> *narrative that may have little to do with*
> *what once transpired and even less to do*
> *with the present moment."*

Pull up grates.

Can I mark up a liberry book?

The pie on the rack on the kitchen table is a homely specimen, bearing no resemblance to the hundreds of effortless, magazine-cover pies she produced —

— 'unlovely' pie —

— perfect pies (apple, cherry, pumpkin, chocolate, strawberry rhubarb, blueberry, lemon meringue ...

Drought yard, burnt brown —

— twiggy hands, like (*Nana's gone to heaven* —

Squirrels —

— pitchforks —

Behind the stack of dessert plates, a bottle of generic coated aspirin tipped over on its side, the seven-day pill container, the blue plastic pill-cutter —

Resolved: cheek zit; sluggish bowels; belly blemishes

Safe in their — Mémère, Pépère, Dad, Mom (room for two more —

— arabesques through the maple, in and out of the birdhouses —

RESTLESSNESS (repetitive motions such as —

Unresolved: fatigue; crippled morning feet; neck lump

Thick leaf pads along the fence bottoms —

Returned: head hair (thinner); pubes (some-ish); leg and underarm hair (sparse); nose hairs; eyelashes (snaily progress)

Final *Black Krim*, roseblush —

Lost: sensation in right armpit and right underarm;
menses

— sliced with a grind of pepper and a sprinkle of Grey
Sea Salt.

Returned: appetite; white count; pink tongue; weight
(nearly one year —

— clover, of which there was an —

Gained: menopause

Halloween — once —

Carpe diem the cloudy, mild afternoon to tidy the garden.

I kneel on the old blue bathmat and clip overgrown
grasses and clumps of brown dead grass from the stone
borders, dirt rectangle and circles where the tomato pots
stood.

Room, at last, to maneuver the mower through, but the
ordeal of dragging it from the garage, up the driveway
staircase, unwinding and winding the long orange —

   COME UP SOONER RATHER THAN —

Zen snipping, clipping blades and straws, one cluster at a
time.

At the base of the emptied pot beneath the matted coir liner, an earthworm writhes, perplexed that her world has been literally rocked.

Tomato roots had thrust their way through the liner, then the drainage holes, and burrowed into the ground —

   ICD9: 197.7 Secondary Malig Neo Liver

I clip dead vines into reasonable lengths, lay them along the fence, my improvised compost, then scatter tomato dirt along this strip, over matted maple leaves and thready basil roots.

BODY TEMPERATURE (increasingly cool to the –

Walkway: one oblivious _Thai_ basil, lush and purple-flowered; a few struggling, straggling _Genovese_ basils; the robust _Giant of Italy_ parsley colony; vigorous thyme and oregano patches; two dangling _Serrano Tampiqueno_; one _Dwarf Siberian_ kale.

Yard wall: lone _Santa Fe_ pepper; mess of green chives; dead daisies; three-quarter eaten kale; anemic, neglected arugula in the far corner.

Gnat-sized insects bombard my face as I clip, disrupting their ecosystem.

Skeletons from trees —

Plastic graves —

Skulls and hands reach out of the earth —

Trick-or-treaters negotiate pitch black sidewalks and
curbstones in a town that cannot afford light.

Fat smiling pumpkins (you were 'Clown', 'Queen',
'Headless Horseman' —

— this may indicate readiness for the final shutdown.

NOVEMBER

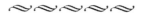

Faux hurricane for fun.

Fifty mile an hour winds strip leaves; swirl debris on lawns and driveways; down branches and twigs from the cemetery into the yard.

More prominent maple skeleton.

Approaching 70°!?

Residual foliage produces a monochrome, rust-orange effect, though individual leaves are comprised of greens, russets, blonds.

Squirrels scavenge the disrupted landscape.

Pointillism?

A plastic bag spins through the driveway and embraces the fire hydrant.

Neurotic blinks of sun and —

UNUSUAL COMMUNICATION: Accept the moment as a beautiful gift.

More dark gray spitting sky, gusts rocking (squeezing words, folding down the tube —

My infusion suite and treatment center were, at least cosmetically, more upscale and shiny than her decrepit, near-bankrupt institution.

USE 4 DROPS SUBLINGUALLY

My phlebotomists found one easily, time and again, even when my arm was blue-purple from extra-curricular inpatient assaults. They drew virtually markless samples, while she came home covered with dark purple wounds, triumphant if the procedure took only "three tries".

SLEEPING (increasing amount of time sleeping —

My biweekly praise and gratitude were deflected; they insisted they were merely doing their —

— uncommunicative or unresponsive —

I was able to drag my IV up and down the gleaming corridor to the bathroom; help myself to peanuts, bad granola bars, endless bottles of (Constipation Wars) water; watch television; read; or close my eyes in my own spacious infusion room.

A year ago *this* —

She was confined to a chair in a row of chairs, flanked by flimsy drapes with no privacy or ability to make a phone call; nowhere to walk; no freedom to even go to the bathroom without being unhooked by a nurse.

A year ago —

Port Follies: my Partially Collapsed Lung vs. her Kinked Tubing

A year ago —

Her <u>three</u> surgical port procedures at two hospitals:
    a) failure
    b) transfer to new site
    c) failure to correct the failure
    d) transfer back to site of original failure
    e) success

My <u>two</u> surgical port procedures at two hospitals:
    a. failure
    b. partially collapsed lung
    c. transfer to Boston for overnight stay
    d. insertion by vascular specialists
    e. success

She promptly contracted both *C-diff* <u>and</u> *VRE*.

— jaw relaxed and mouth slightly —

> "*VRE* have been recovered from bedposts, sheets,
> call buttons, telephones, horizontal surfaces,
> doorknobs, and equipment such as stethoscopes
> and thermometers."

All terracotta to the garage —

> "*Clostridium difficile* is shed in feces, and transfer to
> patients is mainly via the hands of healthcare
> personnel who have touched a contaminated
> surface or —"

Red-orange maple leaves thick on walkway and grass,
26° —

How we could have —

Shocks of red sumac among cemetery golds and greens.

A year ago *this* —

> **<u>Your wound will not open.</u>**

She wore the blonde wig on Thanksgiving.

> — EVEN REASONABLY CONFIDENT YOU WON'T
> COME INTO CONTACT WITH SOMEONE WHO —

My brother drove us to my aunt's in New Hampshire.

Daylight —

We were all clueless that in *ten weeks* —

— dusk, 4:30 PM.

My uncle escorted her gingerly down the wide front steps, across the gravel driveway to the car.

A cool, moist washcloth on the forehead —

We concurred — *a lovely day* — on the long drive home.

Cold blue sunshine —

She'd made her famous *Sally Lunn* rolls; her carrot cake, too.

— eyes fixed on a certain spot —

— my compulsion to hoard all these laxatives, the anti-nausea prescription bottles, the sticks with the blue sponges —

EVERY 4 HOURS AS NEEDED

— knew — did not know — could not have known —

Overnight, half the leaves (calendar —

— bushes trimmed and sculpted around the stones.

Extra glow-green turf in preparation for Veterans Day and the coming holidays (PLEASE – ABSOLUTELY NO FEEDING –

— last *Santa Fe* by the wall, a pair of *Serranos* —

Maple showerfall (inhale, inhale —

Seamless blend with no hint of —

A year ago —

American flags on graves of all the veterans — my father—

Across the path, the matching green fully reseeded, expectant.

Red sumac shocks across the crumbling graves.

I frisbee twigs and small branches back over the wall into the tangled jungle. Both 'chuck den and mound are buried beneath the pruned branches that had brushed the house.

Racket of leaf blowers — rush to —

Abandoned?

A partial solar is invisible —

At Cooks Valley ('since 1705') Farm, wooden stalls of butternut squash; garlic braids from the rafters; fat squat pumpkins —

— chill winds —

Their Cook descendants through the bathroom window, sprouting sumac.

Ladybugs and boxelders scoot up the kitchen screen seeking —

Eliza Cook Sweet, 1816-1822

(I should mention this to them someday.)

Hose on its stand.

Terracotta pots to the garage.

Abundance of greens among the beets and cauliflower; ten varieties of heirloom apples —

Lower leaves shimmer —

I like to sample a new variety every fall. *Mutsu*'s tough, crunchy skin, tart-crisp —

Dewy frost on the long brown grass.

Ida Red, Jonagold, Fuji, Winesap, Spartan —

Photos on the hutch and refrigerator, media console (swing, mid-air, *big straw hat* —

Dead, dead — peppers — basil —

— sera — sera —

Corner kale lives, minus several critter-shorn leaves.

Parsley in patches.

Two more bags of compressed, dark orange maple leaves (one quarter remain?) —

Her black winter coat fits fine, newer than my —

This is a wonderful gift.

A gift of *Clivia miniata* — orange blossoms to anticipate through the coming —

Terracotta to the garage.

— few brown-orange leaves ripple —

Cool windy showers. Maple nearly bare, though woods flush with golds, greens, reds.

Many yards (not this one) still green.

Mould and moss and mushrooms in the long dead —

Mossy cement in the shade of the shed.

A few dozen pale brown leaves along the bottom —

— for a 'healthy' lawn, which I take to mean a deep and thorough rake scrape, enough to upend the earthworms and start the blue jay/sparrow party —

I do try not to bury the odd frantic spider in the leaf bag.

— *sera* — *sera* —

I flick a glow green worm into the grass.

Four more bags of crumbly, showered-upon leaves, a good portion retrieved from the Bermuda Triangle behind the rhododendron.

Pungent, damp leaves compact more easily than the dried, fly-away variety. Breezes spur me to hustle —

My new oncologist presses my bare belly quadrants with her cold hands.

Maybe it won't happen —

(She does apologize for having Raynaud's.)

Cracked graves reveal themselves among the bare twigs and stripped trees.

First flakes mid-November, nothing sticking —

— parsley, between thyme and the last of the —

Whiplash back to 60° —

Boxelder finds herself on the wrong side of the kitchen window above the sink.

Five bags full — browner, less crispy specimens.

Jelly jar to catch, capture, and release just outside the back —

Handful of chewed leaves on the bare frame —

— calendar collage — *on the swing* — *at the beach* — *with the ice cream* —

Labs good with the exception of —

       Maybe —

— a single elevated —

       Maybe —

Vigorous raking aerates clumps of moss in the shadiest corners.

She will see me (yes, small world, knew my mother's oncologist, too, Dr. N—, and his son, who is also going into the family business) in <u>six months</u>.

— incrementally, by pieces of street on the far side now, lights from a neighbor's upstairs windows through the cemetery tree bones.

The pile of pruned branches and trimmings across the burrow entrance has wilted and begun to collapse.

— fastidious, leaves from the beds — mocking green chives —

Nature column in today's paper: "... blue jays gather the acorns from the treetops before they fall to the ground and may be eaten by other wildlife."

What a simple yet ingenious mechanism for rake expansion and contraction.

— *bones? spine?*

"Amazingly, they can fly and carry five small acorns at a time, with three in the throat, one in the mouth, and one in the —"

Changes along your scars?

"During the fall a blue jay will bury and hide thousands of nuts, one at a time, to help sustain through —"

Cold hands in my armpits; fingertips along —

I'm right behind you.

66° sunshine. Everyone rushes outside in thin spring coats.

Flora flummoxed.

BP seems high, even 'white coat'. I retest at home with
her cuff retrieved from under the bathroom sink.

Christmas cacti blooms in the sunporch.

Nearly identical, if slightly worse. A brisker than usual
Resurrection walk to raise heart rate (?)

The *Yellow* (green) *Pears* in the basket refuse to ripen.
Now some shriveling.

Small handful of luncheon arugula.

Three kale leaves from the corner.

OCD retest seated at the kitchen table: 122/81

Daredevil squirrels off the wall — kamikaze staircase —

Highs in the 20s predicted for Thanksgiving week.

— each strand distinct, glistening gray —

Pine needles stab my fingers through the blue cloth
gloves.

Dirty butts at the base of the driveway.

— left clavicle soreness —

Pluck and drop in the brown trash —

Tired, tired, fractured —

Only a year ago *this*, a year ago —

    — LIVE IN THE HEARTS THEY LEAVE BEHIND NEVER —

— year *from now* —

Manicured, leaf-swept Resurrection deserted due to the chilly temps. Four wind-blown laps.

    FOREVER IN OUR HEARTS

Goose poop, whole and smeared, confined to one five-yard arc of roadway.

— a year ago —

— pointed pain in the left —

The dying person might experience varied and mixed —

Pale green *Clivia* buds poised; Christmas cacti half-bloom—

Maple spikes rocking —

Leaves tumbling —

    FOREVER

No evidence of life remains in the grass.

Thanksgiving morning, 22° in New Hampshire.

BREATHING PATTERN CHANGE

A pair of red (!) squirrels shimmy up and down my uncle's bird feeders.

Two — three — four neon orange blooms with reddish stamens.

Six or seven more buds —

— shallow breaths with periods of no breathing (5 to 30 seconds and up to a full —

— brown forsythia leaves and broken branches by the garage door since last week's sweepings —

SEE YOU IN HEAVEN

December

Dusk —

Neighbors weave lights through trees.

Electric candy canes —

Santas on mailboxes —

Wreaths at windows —

Across the street, the reindeer flickers white, head bent
and up again beside the white angel.

Boxes down from the cubbyhole: sleds; cards; bells;
stuffed bears; snowmen candles; centerpieces; crèche; the
ancient plastic wreath for the front door.

Despite my efforts to put decorations in their rightful —
no, not there — historic nooks —

Belongs where?

Listening — straining for —

Who now can corroborate —

Paperwhites arrive. I place the basket of bulbs in the cool
spare bedroom until the roots 'take hold' in some three
weeks, says the booklet.

Three big ducks (geese? pondered the dunderhead) —
two gray with red markings around the bills, one white
— spread their wings, peddling beneath the murk,
loitering at the edges of the pond beside the wood slat
fence.

— mid-60s to high teens —

Fatter, bushier, winter coat chipmunks scour the lawn,
leap the wall, dive-bomb the Bermuda —

Beige lepidopterist-specimen moths paste themselves to
the kitchen screen —

Panic of cars pound the street, mall-bound this gray
Sunday before the ice storm.

— *doesn't belong* —

RESTLESSNESS (repetitive motions such as —

Clivia blooms.

DISORIENTATION (time, place identity)

Jasmine buds.

Cigarette Butt Festival, last of the forsythia branches and assorted leaves on the driveway into one small garbage bag.

Christmas cacti — like popcorn —

Tug the *Paperwhite* bulbs for 'resistance' as per instructions —

Senseless to replace or purchase another —

INCONTINENCE (loss of bladder and/or bowel —

6:44 AM: black driveway — rink hazard —

— entrenched and relocated to sunny sunporch to join her potted pals.

Car — mailbox — lawn —

CONGESTION (gurgling sounds)

The morning's obituary skim yields the father of an elementary schoolmate, now a radiologist.

WHO ARRANGE ME 'PRECISELY' ON THE TABLE
IN CHRIST-LIKE POSITION, FOR A ROUGHLY TEN
MINUTE ZAPPING, AS A GIANT PLATE WHIRS AND
GRINDS UP AND DOWN AND AROUND.

(She used to play the violin, or I could be hallucinating?)

Cannellini beans bubble on the stove — cold drear —

I'M AFRAID I HAVE VERY LITTLE —

I said I *heard her voice in my — instructing —*

She was equivocal, though after consulting with
colleagues came down a bit more firmly on Team Nuke.

Christmas bells looped on the back doorknob tinkle
coming and going.

— (quantifiable 'mortality benefit' —

— tinkle tones —

> "The absolute overall survival benefit at 5 and 10
> years was relatively small (1.6 to 3.3%), but the
> available survival curves indicate that a larger
> benefit may occur with longer follow-up."
>
> *Radiation Oncology*: 2013, 8:267

— supine in a machine the size of a small tank, likely
approaching, if not already surpassing obsolescence —

Maybe —

A couple of times over my treatment the behemoth was deemed out of commission like a faulty transmission; my daily appointment was pushed forward.

Laws of Inertia —

After my final zap, the (inexplicable) number 33, the nice technicians emerged from the glass booth and presented me with a 'diploma' and a balloon.

Palpitations (heart muscle —

I pitied their dreary, claustrophobic, radioactive jobs, and imagined our 30-second party was as much for them as for me.

— skull fermentation — squeeze —

We all grinned and shook hands and pretended we'd see each other again.

Heart attack?

Am I —

— about heart attacks — *no* —

Rain gems on maple branches —

Poinsettias, etc.

A year ago *this*, a year ago —

— looped on the doorknob —

Poinsettias on so many graves.

— of the tabletop Christmas 'tree', a balsam arrangement smelling absolutely —

Christmas baskets and wreaths.

— revolving car doors, none lingering in the cold —

— year ago —

Accelerated heartbeat —

— a year ago —

Indifference to suggested (1) bone density
(2) colonoscopy (3) flu shot (4) tetanus

SPIRITUAL AND EMOTIONAL

(5) grief counselor

Reynolds Pond frozen over.

Ice melt (ineffective) along the bottom of the driveway for the mail carrier to deliver the latest TLC catalog of beanies, turbans, wigs, and head scarves addressed to her ghost.

Six fat geese-ducks in and near the water hole behind the chain-link and wood slat fences.

Fresh Baker Creek catalog, glossy heirlooms (gardener 'crack' —

A new fellow, black dashed with white, paddles the icy—

Tabletop tree decorated.

Needles and garland glitter —

Plug in — !!

— black ice over 95% of the driveway. I leave the newspaper where it fell.

Impassable; wind chill of 8° —

— even beneath a pair called 'Thinsulate' invite semi-frost-bite —

Chink-chink-chank — neighbors hack ice — or pick coal —

Ray plows me out with his new old pickup.

Paper retrieved; headline: *Breast Cancer Study blah blah... blah...*

Moonglow snow.

... blah blah ...

More snow.

7°.

Few, if any, bother to slow down along the hazard-slick major road.

Polar desert through the window.

... blah ... May Alter ... blah blah... Treatment ... blah blah...

The prospect of tackling a Bûche de Noël for the first time tempts, but all in all too —

(Two houses down a car bangs into a mother turning into her driveway.)

Do this that don't do this or that —

I'm right behind you.

Three, four, five sparrows in the maple, and one more pokes her head through the hole in the house.

"*We don't* (have no idea) *really —*"

Cardinal flame against the snow.

— for the company —

Dirty snow crusts ringed with twig and leaf debris; pale gold grass.

Next year — next —

"Save some seeds each year!"

(The rogue potatoes are a big hit.)

" — you will help preserve your heritage — "

Second Christmas miracle; births of cream-colored
jasmine and luminous *Paperwhites* —

Tears on my (her) blue sweater, the edges of my loaded
Plate of Many Colors.

— so many Bicycle decks stashed around the house, the
hutch, her bureau.

Family photo —

I wrap them as presents to the 'card sharp' grandkids, one
seal-broken, well-worn, Pitch-exhausted deck apiece —
'from Grandma' —

Palpitations in the cold, at rest —

She and my father taught the five of them how to play.

Constant cold in the extremities.

*"Screaming-hot peppers turn a rainbow of
vibrant — "*

'Hothouse' perfume in the cold, cold sunporch —

I hold my hands under water to warm them.

(1) *Paperwhites* two feet tall, in a green metal hoop (2) pot of jasmine —

Moonbeam —

— cacti wither and drop —

— blizzard approaches, a foot or more —

> " — *purple, cream, yellow, orange to red* — "

The neighbor's Christmas Pomeranian cavorts with his sister pug before the snow arrives.

BE WELL.

JANUARY

"Presently the rude Real burst coarsely in ..."

CHARLOTTE BRONTË, <u>VILLETTE</u>

I gather the balance into a paper bag and scatter the still fragrant branches beneath the lilac, and a few into the Bermuda —

— jingle bells on doorknob —

— ancient plastic wreath —

— ceramic crèche figurines and cardboard stable —

— stuffed snowmen —

— Santas (made in Japan! —

— angels —

— Three Wise —

— tall red candles —

Vacuum *pittle-pittle* balsam needles —

Silence, but for the —

"Big Clock, Lil' Clock" — odd quarter hours —

Cracked skin and cracked lips (half-full tubes of hand
and heel cream —

— *swing and straw hat* on the wall beside the telephone —

-21° —

4:14 AM.

— *sera — sera —*

4:48 AM.

Ray crosses the street in the pitch black and plows the
driveway mess into a tidy 8' mountain.

... cotton sports socks under black knee-highs under
vintage brown wool (scratchy horsehair?) 'skating' socks
(knit by obscure Quebecois antecedents on their mystery
farm?) from the grab bag in the hallway closet, wedged
into her old waterproof snow boots; two pairs of gloves
inside vintage brown (Quebecois) wool mittens; gray
long-johns under thick green corduroys; black turtleneck;
blue sweater; purple flotation-device winter coat; red
inner scarf; black ski hat; maroon outer scarf; hood pulled
tight with a black rubber cord ...

Wind, winds —

I rush to clear car, steps, garage door, mailman's walkway and mailbox (hypothermic right toes, wedged in boot —

— *Chill — then Stupor —*

— even in the house, compulsory fingerless gloves with the tops cut —

Mounting mounds against the wall, stagger on the stairs (toes — foot — feet —

— *Chill — then —*

I roll back sock layers to excavate super red toes — bad sign? good?

— *Ceremonious —*

(I can stand — walk — feel — a little —

Maybe it won't —

Ramrod *Paperwhite* in the cold, cold —

Orchid bloom — impervious —

Weakest sun melts roof and hood, random streaks across the driveway.

Baker Creek 'Seed-uction' —

The fingerless gloves shed purple thread crumbs across bedspread and floor.

A year ago *this* —

Before rehab discharge could be granted an 'assistive device kit' had to be ordered from a local medical device company — the 'Reacher' – the shoe horn – the sock thing — and a contractor hired (far more difficult than anticipated) to install a pair of grab bars in the shower.

A year ago —

One year ago —

DISORIENTATION (time, place identity)

In the stuffy gym of wheelchair oldsters she plodded up and down a small incline with the aid of her new walker.

A year ago —

The doctor joked (had he been joking?) that the worrisome symptoms might be treated by eating Dorritos.

— foreseen, had we only —

A year ago —

"... reduce intake of water ..."

The three of us smiled, straining to digest this remedy.

"... decreased consciousness, hallucinations or coma, brain herniation, or death ..."

One year ago —

Identify yourself by name before you speak.

He soon disappeared and was neither seen nor heard from again.

We tried on our own to research this because the nursing home staff couldn't begin to —

— year ago *that* —

— *Ceremonious, like Tombs* —

Some months later, his name surfaced in the local newspaper for malfeasance, delivering "care below accepted minimal standards ..."

Paperwhite perfume —

Dried, dried, dried, cracked —

Recognizing Signs & Symptoms

Snowmelt weeps down the windows.

— Chill — then —

I dreamt the lilac died, shorn off its roots in the blizzard.

Saturday-deserted.

Not the wind chill but my cripple-boots, constricted
under layers of scratchy, Quebecois horsehair socks, force
me to abort my walk after two short laps.

Untouched snow against the graves; bowls of slope and
ridge down to bare grass where winds have chiseled
out—

White desert.

— year ago —

White moon.

> *Until the Moss had reached our lips —*
> *And covered up — Our names —*

Single white strand from the flowered fabric chair.

Hyacinths, not *daffodils* (Bette on her knees with a trowel—

No footprints or tracks in the snow yard; no birds in the
maple or houses.

"I HAVE BEEN SAVING THIS CARD FOR <u>YEARS</u>—"

Everything snowballed, though the visiting nurse had declared her vitals 'fine'.

I remained twilight-awake on the couch all night, stumbling to her bedside on some ten or so occasions when I heard moaning or the heavy clang of walker wheels as she made her way to the bathroom.

— contorted in what seemed like rigor mortis, hands clenched like claws —

No, not in pain, she said.

I guided her stiff arms, her shoulders gently back flat to the bed.

Around 6:00 AM I heard the now familiar thud of body against wooden floor. In my rush down the hall, I wrenched an ankle and fell, fluttering out of consciousness, but was able to drag myself over to her now vacated bed and rest for some thirty long seconds.

I watched her from above.

As soon as my head cleared I lifted her to an upright position, leaned her back against the side of the bed and told her not to move.

She lapsed at once into a snoring, chin-on-chest coma.

For the third time in ten months, the EMTs arrived, mercifully, assessed her vitals, strapped her to a stretcher—

Attending Salt & Pepper barked at me for loitering near the nurses' station as I tried to relay incrementally recalled medical history.

I sat in a vinyl chair at the foot of her cot to doze across my forearm.

Every so often she would rouse and urge me to go home, I *looked so tired*.

Many hours passed.

Many hours.

Hours.

Salt & Pepper took me aside and said the head scan showed *no metastasis*, that the only lab finding was *low sodium*.

A social worker came to help us arrange —

— of lucidity, we managed to eliminate some of the reputed worst facilities, but her preferences were naturally booked and we were pushed through the Looking Glass into the — Nursing Home, where we met the cartoon Dr. —.

He squatted to dispense his wisdom in the hot double room while the deaf crone roommate glided to and from her bed-residence by the window.

Dorritos! (we smiled and nodded, drugged chimps—

Twenty-four, thirty-six hours of stroke-like conversation and drift—

Clivia petals to the maroon flowered bench —

— dreams; slow walker-walk down the corridor to the 'rec' room; needle-taped port, *still* accessed —

— orchid buds —

— bad lemon pudding; white gauze; multiple trips to the nurses' station (excuses, bewilderment, defensiveness as to why the needle in her clavicle should be attended to); care not to alienate the crew who held her life literally in their hands the many hours we could not be —

<u>Sixty hours</u> sum 'captivity'.

I chip away at the snow piles, hard-packed slicks at the base of the driveway, with the lousy shovel before the sleet —

... jumbo tub of Quaker Oats; box of incandescent lightbulbs; plastic bag of assorted screwdrivers; converter plugs, box cutters, electrical ...

A year ago —

— eyes fixed on a certain spot, no blinking —

Baker Creek fantasy, many 'arable acres': mosaic of sunflowers, basils, peppers —

How soon to seed-start? not as ignorant; still very ignorant —

Her surgeon tapped his fingers on her chest, scalp and back — *here* and *here* and *here.*

I trailed him to the ER nurses station.

Six months, he said.

So why, why necessary to roll her in a blanket in a stretcher in February, transfer across town to endure hours of additional medical —

I nodded — nodded.

(We had *seven days*.)

— red, yellow, green, pink, striped, purple, blush tomatoes —

I'm right behind —

I kept the wooden, accordion-playing angel, the size of my thumbnail, on the desk.

Maybe it won't —

The flab beneath my right arm feels puffier some days than —

Scraping and shaving the driveway with the Island of Misfit shovels: (1) unwieldy yellow clunker that refuses to release the snow (2) crumbling green plastic scoop with bites taken out of the bottom (3) weird 'pusher' —

— race, race the coming —

— sera — sera —

No.

Balmy rebound to the 50s, another snow-eater, down to bare grass; rapid shrinkage of filthy pile beneath the forsythia.

Four laps in unseasonable warmth and fog.

Water swamps some graves. Many Christmas decorations removed.

> *" — almost a cult following among tomato connoisseurs —"*

American flags on stones, leftover from Veterans Day? Greenish algae creeps downward, obscuring Mémère's name and Pépère's name, not —

"— distinctive, sweet and smoky —"

— pea-sized welt (?) above my left eyebrow —

Maybe —

— mirror, mirror (no reddening —

Pleas to renew her subscriptions: *Martha Stewart Living; Cooking Light; Vanity Fair*

Balm before tonight's Arctic —

Please don't leave us.

Tired — tired —

NO MORE THAN A MONTH, BUT WE SUSPECT—

— dissipates in the night (might as easily —

Tired — tired — freeze — thaw —

HOSPICE PEOPLE HELPING TO KEEP HER —

Firemen spring from their truck and snow blow a path to the hydrant.

Stinging pinpoints in the armpit (sometimes the *grossness* of looking in the mirror —

Morning snowdust, rewhiting yard; driveway; steps.

Birdhouse askew, rope-snapped (too frigid to set right).

— parsley and kale under snow cover; brown rosemary—

Opaque gray ice.

(Vermont has passed a Patient Choice and Control at End of Life Act.)

Eight geese-ducks, four elders and four youngers, bask in the frost behind the chain link and wood slat —

— puffiness — tiredness —

I prune the Christmas cacti, halving its sprawl.

Shriveled brown rosemary —

Toss greens in the Bermuda Triangle?

Chapped hands —

Pruned jasmine basket —

　　　　"Sow as a spring crop where summers —"

Green sprawl of *Clivia* —

Succession of tires on the sleety (childhood skating on frozen —

— sleety freezing (white skate into black water —

SADLY THE NEWS IS VERY BAD.

Seven men surround a grave, heads bent in the rain.

ANYONE WHO WANTS TO SEE HER SHOULD NOT
WAIT —

— unable to retie the cord, rain sheeting down my face.

Amaryllis — single bulb in white wicker —

I place the house on the ground at the base of the maple.

Never assume the person <u>cannot</u> —

I do secure the cord (albeit slightly lopsided —

"... residents who are suffering from an incurable and
irreversible ..."

Birdhouses rock in the breeze.

— quarter hour — half hour echo —

— on the return of the sparrows in the —

Jasmine petals on frosted glass —

Paperwhites —

Rearrange Spanish moss?

"Vigorous vines give large yields —"

Fat fluff snow feathers —

A year ago —

— gray sky; walkway steps and driveway —

If you are part of the final inner circle of support, the person needs your affirmation —

Foot of fresh —

More cherry tomatoes, exotic striped ones, green and yellow and gold, def 'indeterminate' —

Maybe sunflowers along the wall.

Mesclun, lettuce, leeks, mustards "do well in partial shade", so may rethink the fence row?

Happy Birthday, VW.

— affirmation, support, and permission —

Will Mr. W see his shadow.

Paperwhite pops among the spent —

Maybe —

(Description is good for the soul, says Ole Golly.)

I'd never thought of gardens in that way.

Flurry of robins and a blue jay comb the brown lawn for treasures.

Maple of sparrows (three houses *ocupada*) shivers in the cold.

FEBRUARY

"Who are we? What are we doing? —
My eyes take big gulps of Night's black wine."

HÉLÈNE CIXOUS, FIRST DAYS OF THE YEAR

Beak tips — beaks — babies — from each of the snow-
covered —

Perfect buffet for Tan Bunny.

"Makes pretty pickles and salsa."

Snowdust blasts my double-scarved face as I clear
windshield and barrels, steps and walkway —

(Ah, the mystery tomato pole was the other half of the
'snow rake'.)

Piano leg icicles from the eaves —

On the physical level —

Sparrows leap to snowless limbs.

1 yellow wedding band

Jar a boxelder paralyzed on the white curtain.

A widower clears a grave with a yellow shovel.

Release into snow.

— camouflaged, delicacies in the forsythia branches —

Powdery snow-fog in wide bands across my path, lap
number four —

Blue birds? 'Scrubs'? at the neighbor's feeder —

Final week for decorations, wreaths on graves.

Right scar soreness. Extra puffy —

Mirror, mirror —

Hold your loved one's —

Rotate toward the light —

Whole body vibrations —

Diagonal squirrel tracks beneath the fence by the maple,
breaking the neighbor's unbroken —

— thrumming skull — dry cough —

I tucked her in.

— thrumming (cars bouncing potholes? —

She said *you're a wonderful* —

— granola cinnamon up the stairs —

— thrumming —

Speak gently.

Piano legs to the pavement —

Three fat (obese) geese-ducks stroll the pond.

We intercepted steaming, lumberjack-portioned slop on trays just outside the room. I brought her slices of green apple from home, a few bites of —

Dr. N— came on Saturday, in his civilian clothes, to tell us what we already knew.

You have a very sad job, she said.

Somebody's got to do it.

At the door he turned back to embrace her bedside —

OBIT ON WEDNESDAY. BURIAL AT
RESURRECTION CEMETERY.

Four sets of four chimes —

GETTING VERY SLIPPERY HERE ALTHOUGH
LITTLE ACCUMULATION THUS FAR.

... on the hour, quarter hour ...

*"... GRIEF IS SUCH A MYSTERIOUS THING, AND
NO ONE KNOWS —"*

**SAYING GOODBYE: It may be as simple as saying I love
you.**

ACKNOWLEDGEMENTS

Enormous gratitude to my siblings for their encouragement, phone calls and visits, for making hospital, clinic and pharmacy runs, for walking beside me as I lurched along, never letting me fall.

Thanks to Laura for the meticulous notes; John, Johnny, Richard, Michel and Cynthia for their steady support; nieces and nephews whose presence was always a cheerful distraction; my large extended family, with shout-outs to Bill, Roger, Richard, Benny and Charlotte, who pitched in during some difficult days; and numerous friends near and far.

Everyone should have such wonderful neighbors: Kathy, Val, Ray and Dawn.

Margaret, Zoe and Marie sustained me across the miles, more than they know.

For the doctors, nurses and professionals, the medical, clinical and support staff who cared for me and my mother, and daily toil under some of the most stressful conditions imaginable, I am indebted. Thank you.

So many people have fortified me on this journey, but I would be remiss if I did not single out in particular the heroic contributions of my aunt Jeanne, who was with us both every step of the way. She is a rock star.